Health and Welfare of ART Children

REPRODUCTIVE MEDICINE & ASSISTED REPRODUCTIVE
TECHNIQUES SERIES

Series Editors

David K Gardner DPhil
Colorado Center for Reproductive Medicine, Englewood, CO, USA

Jan Gerris MD PhD
Professor of Gynecology, University Hospital Ghent, Ghent, Belgium

Zeev Shoham MD
Director, Infertility Unit, Kaplan Hospital, Rehovot, Israel

Forthcoming Titles

1. Gerris, Delvigne and Olivennes: Ovarian Hyperstimulation Syndrome
2. Sutcliffe: Health and Welfare of ART Children
3. Keck, Tempfer and Hugues: Conservative Infertility Management
4. Pellicer and Simón: Stem Cells in Reproductive Medicine
5. Tan, Chian and Buckett: In-vitro Maturation of Human Oocytes
6. Elder and Cohen: Human Embryo Evaluation and Selection
7. Tucker and Liebermann: Vitrification in Assisted Reproduction

Health and Welfare of ART Children

Edited by

Alastair G Sutcliffe MD MRCP FRCPCH
Senior Lecturer in Child Health (Honorary Consultant)
Royal Free and University College Medical School
University College London
London
UK

informa
healthcare

First published in 2006 by Informa Healthcare, Telephone House, 69-77 Paul Street, London EC2A 4LQ, UK.

Simultaneously published in the USA by Informa Healthcare, 52 Vanderbilt Avenue, 7th Floor, New York, NY 10017, USA.

Informa Healthcare is a trading division of Informa UK Ltd. Registered Office: 37–41 Mortimer Street, London W1T 3JH, UK. Registered in England and Wales number 1072954.

A CIP record for this book is available from the British Library.

Library of Congress Cataloging-in-Publication Data available on application

ISBN-13: 9780415379304

Orders may be sent to: Informa Healthcare, Sheepen Place, Colchester, Essex CO3 3LP, UK
Telephone: +44 (0)20 7017 5540
Email: CSDhealthcarebooks@informa.com
Website: http://informahealthcarebooks.com/

For corporate sales please contact: CorporateBooksIHC@informa.com
For foreign rights please contact: RightsIHC@informa.com
For reprint permissions please contact: PermissionsIHC@informa.com

Contents

Contributors

Jacqueline Barnes MSc PhD
Professor of Psychology, Institute for the Study of Children, Families and Social Issues, Birkbeck College, University of London, London, UK

Christina Bergh MD PhD
Professor, Reproductive Medicine, Institute of Clinical Sciences, Sahlgrenska Academy and University Hospital, Göteborg, Sweden

Carol Bower MBBS MSc PhD FAFPHM
Senior Principal Research Fellow and Clinical Professor, Telethon Institute for Child Health Research, University of Western Australia, West Perth, WA, Australia

Elizabeth Bryan MD FRCP FRCPCH
Consultant Paediatrician and Medical Consultant, Multiple Births Foundation, Queen Charlotte's and Chelsea Hospital, London, UK

Jane Denton RGN RM
Director, Multiple Births Foundation, Queen Charlotte's and Chelsea Hospital, London, UK

Michèle Hansen BSc MPH
Project Officer, Telethon Institute for Child Health Research, University of Western Australia, West Perth, WA, Australia

Jennifer J Kurinczuk BSc MBChB MSc MD FFPH FAFPHM
Consultant Clinical Epidemiologist, National Perinatal Epidemiology Unit, University of Oxford, Oxford, UK

Vic Larcher BA MB BChir MA FRCP FRCPCH
Consultant in Paediatrics and Clinical Ethics, Great Ormond Street
Hospital, London, UK

Annika K Ludwig MD
Gynaecologist and Obstetrician, Department of Gynaecology and
Obstetrics, University of Schleswig-Holstein, Lübeck, Germany

Joe Leigh Simpson MD
Ernst W Bertner Chairman and Professor, Department of Obstetrics and
Gynecology, Baylor College of Medicine, Houston, TX, USA

Alastair G Sutcliffe MD MRCP FRCPCH
Senior Lecturer in Child Health (Honorary Consultant), Royal Free and
University College Medical School, University College London, London,
UK

Ulla-Britt Wennerholm MD PhD
Associate Professor, Department of Obstetrics, Institute of Clinical
Sciences, Sahlgrenska Academy and University Hospital, Göteborg,
Sweden

To my wife Nurhan and my children Elâ, Jan and Papatya,
by whom my life is infinitely enriched

Preface

The second edition of *IVF Children: the First Generation* has a new title. This partly reflects the fact that the first generation of IVF children are now growing up and more importantly that this book is intended to be less personal and more systematic in the way that it covers the subject. For this I am indebted to the experts who I have invited to write the majority of the chapters in this book, whilst maintaining a personal touch within the chapters that I have written myself.

The subject of bias is important in science and particularly medical science. It has been said by one cynic that there is nothing more indignant than a vested interest manifesting as a moral crusade. Throughout the book there are descriptions of the bases on which the chapters are written (in terms of the underlying scientific reports). An attempt has been made to be as accurate as possible whilst not drawing false conclusions where the evidence is not supportive. The subject of assisted conception and the health of children is constantly in the public eye. I hope that some members of the public will enjoy reading this book, although it is principally aimed at medical scientists, fertility specialists, fertility nurses and all those involved with assisted conception. As a pediatrician with no personal stake in assisted conception (apart from having performed a number of research projects in this area), I hope to be as neutral as possible in describing the outcomes, whilst leaning towards the positive as is my general attitude towards the care of children and their families.

It is hoped that the book will provide a useful source of information in one place for those who wish to have a reference. This is a changing field, which is reflected in the fact that this book required updating in such a short space of time. I trust you will enjoy reading it. In some chapters there is a degree of overlap between the topics. This is inevitable because many aspects of outcome can blur into one another, and I consider that it would have been presumptuous to edit out the hard work of some of the co-authors in order to avoid small overlaps. Indeed, the different interpretation of the data, where there is any, will reflect the uncertainties in this area of knowledge and also the different styles and opinions of the individuals who have co-authored this book, and with whom it has been a privilege to work.

Alastair G Sutcliffe
University College London

Chapter 1

Problems in assessing pediatric outcome of ART

Joe Leigh Simpson

By way of introduction to this book, we need to consider the context concerning some aspects of assisted reproductive technology (ART) children's health and welfare. This book reviews the studies of children conceived after various types of ART and discusses these findings in the context of the three categories below.

(1) Presence or absence of major congenital anomalies in children resulting from successful ART;

(2) Growth and neurodevelopmental wellbeing in ART children;

(3) Family relationships that may be altered as a result of the birth of a child from ART.

In this first chapter difficulties in interpreting studies addressing these various outcomes are considered. From the pediatric perspective the outcome of ART can be considered in each of several perspectives.

ETIOLOGY OF CONGENITAL ANOMALIES (BIRTH DEFECTS)

Approximately 3% of liveborn infants have a major congenital anomaly. About one-half of these anomalies are detected at birth; the remainder become evident later in childhood or, less often, adulthood. Factors identified as causing malformations usually prove to be genetic. Non-genetic factors exist but are recognized far less often. The role of genetic factors in causing abnormal development is underscored by 50% of first-trimester spontaneous abortions and 5% of stillborn infants showing chromosomal abnormalities.

Causes of birth defects

Abnormal development may be considered in terms of several etiologic categories: chromosomal abnormalities; single-gene (or Mendelian) disorders; polygenic/multifactorial disorders, resulting from cumulative effects of more than one gene, possibly interacting with environmental factors; and teratogenic disorders, caused by exposure to exogenous factors (e.g. drugs) that deleteriously affect an embryo otherwise destined to develop normally.

Based on surveys of more than 50 000 liveborn neonates, the incidence of chromosomal aberrations is 1 in 160. Approximately half are autosomal abnormalities and half involve sex chromosomes.

Approximately 1% of liveborns are phenotypically abnormal as a result of a single-gene mutation. Several thousand single-gene (Mendelian) disorders have been recognized, and many more are suspected. Even the most common Mendelian disorders (cystic fibrosis in whites, sickle cell anemia in blacks, β-thalassemia in Greeks and Italians, α-thalassemia in Southeast Asians, Tay–Sachs disease in Ashkenazi Jews) are individually rare.

Another 1% of neonates are abnormal but possess a normal chromosomal complement and have not undergone mutation at a single genetic locus. It can be deduced that several different genes are involved (polygenic/multifactorial inheritance). Disorders in this category include most common malformations limited to a single organ system. These include hydrocephaly, anencephaly and spina bifida (neural tube defects), cleft lip, cleft palate, most cardiac defects and club foot. After the birth of one child with such anomalies, the recurrence risk in subsequent progeny is usually 1–5%. This is less than would be expected if only a single gene were responsible, but far greater than expected for the general population (0.1% or less). Recurrence risks are also 1–5% for offspring of affected patients. That recurrence risks are similar for both siblings and offspring excludes environmental causes as the sole etiologic factor, because households in different generations would not be exposed plausibly to the same teratogen. Further excluding environmental factors as sole etiologic agents are observations that monozygotic twins are much more often similarly affected than are dizygotic twins, despite both types of twins sharing a common intrauterine environment.

PREGNANCY LOSSES IN IVF/ART

The frequency of spontaneous abortion is usually considered to be increased following *in vitro* fertilization (IVF). On the other hand, pregnancy in IVF is diagnosed earlier than in natural conceptions. Figures from the Human Fertilisation and Embryology Authority (HFEA)[1] of the UK suggest that abortion rates in IVF are similar to those of the general population. Although abortion in ART pregnancies is assumed to be the result of hormonal imbalances adversely affecting implantation, an increased abortion rate is of concern, because 50–60% of clinically recognized spontaneous abortions show chromosomal abnormalities. Cytogenetic abnormalities in ART could be, albeit unlikely, the explanation for the increased abortion rate. If chromosomal abnormalities contribute to the increased abortion rate, a corollary is that an increased risk would also exist for ART liveborns.

ANOMALIES ASSOCIATED WITH CONVENTIONAL IVF

That congenital anomalies could be increased in ART pregnancies is plausible for several reasons:

(1) Selective mechanisms operating *in vivo* against morphologically abnormal sperm might not be comparably operative *in vitro*;

(2) An altered hormonal milieu *in vitro* may predispose to damage during meiosis or mitosis and, hence, cause chromosomal aneuploidy;

(3) Point mutations could result from the various chemical exposures inherent in extracorporeal fertilization.

Although surveys and registries have been set up to monitor the rate of anomalies, a recurrent pitfall is that comparisons are typically to outcomes recorded in general population registries of birth defects. The proper comparison group would be infertile women not requiring ART. Obviously this is an impossible request.

Spuriously increased rates

More rigorous surveillance

Examination of neonates born following ART is often more rigorous than that following conventional pregnancy (controls). This well-meaning medical surveillance can be scientifically misleading. Anomalies such as small umbilical hernias, pigmented skin lesions and accessory auricles would not necessarily be recorded in a registry of birth defects in the general population. The disparate rates between centers underscore the lack of consistent criteria and data recording. Examples of more vigorous surveillance for ART pregnancies include the UK Medical Research Council surveillance[1]. This surveillance recorded many anomalies not usually detected in neonatal surveys, such as mild hypospadias and undescended testes. A better comparison might involve a prospective study that takes into account differing standards of record keeping.

Increased ultrasound surveillance

Another assessment bias potentially yielding spuriously increased rates for ART children reflects the more frequent and more detailed ultrasound scans during these pregnancies. For example, in the 1990 American Fertility Society/Society for Assisted Reproductive Technology (AFS/SART) cohort[2], recorded anomalies included periventricular cyst, hydronephrosis and unilateral kidney agenesis. None would have been detected strictly on the basis of physical examination.

Extended surveillance period

A final source of bias arises if assessments continue to be performed on ART children after the early neonatal period. A longer surveillance period contributes to ascertainment incompatibility with normal birth registries, continuing to add anomalies to a list that is effectively closed in a standard registry. An example is inclusion of pyloric stenosis.

Spuriously decreased rates

Failure to look systematically for congenital abnormalities

This is the converse of more rigorous examination leading to a spurious increased rate. Here the bias is less rigorous examination leading to decreased anomaly rates. A decreased anomaly rate might not be appreciated if ART centers failed to assess children systematically for congenital anomalies. Review of hospital case notes would be a poor way of ascertaining anomalies. Casual surveillance probably explains the low anomaly rate recorded in certain surveys, for example 0.7% in Greek cases recorded by Cohen et al.[3] or 0.9% in the 1990 AFS/SART cohort[2]. Failure to search systematically for anomalies is a valid concern in almost all ART cohorts, with a few notable exceptions such as the small IVF case–control study of

Morin and et al.[4] and the intracytoplasmic sperm injection (ICSI) cohort in Brussels[5].

Incomplete follow-up

Another pitfall resulting in spuriously low anomaly rates arises whenever a significant proportion of a given sample is lost to follow-up. One cannot assume that cases lost to follow-up are comparable to cases remaining for analysis. Women lost to follow-up who have experienced a bad outcome (pregnancy loss or birth of an anomalous infant) may resent the invasion of privacy or in some way blame an ART center and, hence, fail to respond to requests for follow-up. Thus, the anomaly rate would be spuriously decreased.

Conversely, women lost to follow-up might not wish to be troubled because their children are healthy and because no personal benefit seems to accrue from participating in a research protocol. They further wish to be considered 'normal', perhaps not wishing to divulge their prior ART in order to avoid perceived stigmatization. The net effect would be a spuriously increased anomaly rate following ART because some normal outcomes would be excluded.

If only a small proportion of cases from a large cohort were lost to follow-up, the remaining subjects could reasonably be assumed to be representative. However, this assumption is not necessarily valid when the outcome sought is infrequent or when a relatively high proportion of cases is lost to follow-up. In ART surveillance the number of cases lost to follow-up may be several-fold greater than the background 4–5% anomaly rate. For example, in the 1998 AFS/SART report[6], 58 anomalies were reported in 3873 babies (1.5%), yet 447 of the babies were lost to follow-up (11.5%). If even 10% of the 447 lost cases were anomalous, overall anomaly rates would have risen to 2.7%. In the most recent HFEA report[1] it was claimed that only 0.8% of all children born from IVF were born with an abnormality. This figure was obtained by relying on centers recording and reporting this information. However, often children are born far from their fertility treatment center, diminishing the likelihood of obtaining valid outcome data.

Inconsistent inclusions and exclusions

Another common methodological pitfall in ART surveillance is pooling anomalies in neonates with anomalies in abortuses (spontaneous or induced). Birth defect registries do not record anomalies in abortuses, induced or spontaneous. Yet the 0.6% rate of chromosomal abnormalities in newborn infants is far less than is found in induced abortuses of 5–12 weeks' gestational age[7], and one-hundredth that found in spontaneous abortuses. The natural history of chromosomal (and other etiologies of birth defects) abnormalities also varies. Considerably fewer than half the trisomy 18 cases detected at amniocentesis survive until birth, whereas two-thirds of trisomy 21 cases survive. Pooling anomalies identified during prenatal cytogenetic surveillance (chorionic villus sampling, amniocentesis) with those detected at birth would thus yield data not comparable to the liveborn general population, although theoretically this would provide more complete outcome data. However, there would be no comparable cohort in the normal population for comparison.

Lack of a proper comparison group

Whether assessing pregnancy losses or congenital anomalies, the major underlying concern is that the ART population is not comparable to the general population. It is not possible to generate the desired two companion groups: infertile couples who become pregnant without ART versus fertile couples randomized to ART despite not needing it. Moreover, the underlying infertility that necessitated ART may be due to factors that also increase the rate of pregnancy loss or anomalies in the children. The underlying cause of infertility could be genetic and also pleiotropic, thus placing offspring at increased a priori risk. An obvious example exists in pregnancies conceived using ICSI necessitated by oligozoospermic men who lack the Y chromosome DAZ (Deleted in AZoospermia) locus. Such azoospermic men with Y deletions *must* transmit the deleted Y to all *male* children, who will also be azoospermic or oligozoospermic.

An achievable comparison group, albeit still not ideal, might be subfertile couples requiring infertility treatment (e.g. ovulation indication but neither IVF nor ICSI). Few such data exist, but this would at least provide comparison to a subfertile sample.

ART couples differ from couples in the general population in other ways. Frequency and severity of past illnesses are not necessarily comparable. Infections producing tubal occlusion could persist in a chronic pathologic condition. Women undergoing ART are usually older than women conceiving naturally (mean age about 27 or 28 years)[8]. In the UK this is about 33 years[9]. Paternal age is also commensurably increased. Advanced maternal age is associated with increased risk of pregnancy loss[10,11] and liveborn aneuploidy[12,13]. Advanced paternal age is associated with *de novo* Mendelian mutations[13–15].

Women undergoing ART also differ from women in the general population with respect to potential confounding variables such as maternal toxin exposure and nutrition. The higher maternal age in women undergoing ART places these women at increased cumulative risk compared with women in the general population. However, their contemporary exposures to toxins such as alcohol and cigarettes are usually lower. The aggregate effect of these contradictory trends is uncertain.

In conclusion, underlying genetic or other medical problems may not only explain the infertility that caused a couple to seek ART, but place their children at increased risk irrespective of the manner by which pregnancy was achieved – natural or ART.

GROWTH AND NEURODEVELOPMENTAL WELLBEING

Difficulty exists in enticing ART families achieving a successful outcome to return for follow-up assessment of their child's postnatal growth and development. Inquiries by the IVF clinic for follow-up are usually initially welcomed by families. 'Why didn't they contact us sooner?' The salutary experience benefits from a 'halo effect' ('They gave us our child'). However, after several months to perhaps 1 or 2 years, ART couples increasingly wish to 'become normal', even conveniently forgetting that ART was required. They understandably do not wish to stigmatize their child.

Validity of follow-up studies becomes diminished as sample size becomes unrepresentative. Studies are further weakened by the absence of a true control group. This is analogous to the problem discussed previously with respect to congenital anomalies. Identifying a control group is additionally difficult because many families with children from ART are by their very nature 'winners' in an exacting and psychologically stressful process. In many investigations this selective advantage can be addressed by selecting a sibling control, but for obvious reasons this is not possible.

Neurodevelopmentally, ART children experience both positive and negative influences on their wellbeing. On the 'downside' they are often born prematurely with a lower mean birth weight. Their mothers are older and more likely to have medical complications of pregnancy. On the 'upside' they are often born to families with greater means and higher socioeconomic status. It is these factors that allowed their families to pay for ART treatment in the first place.

The aphorism that 'growth is a bioassay of wellbeing' is important in considering the significance of the health of a child. Assessing growth should be simpler than assessing development, because national growth parameters exist. Providing that valid account is taken of parental heights, and providing that measurements are standardized and serial, long-term growth effects on the ART-conceived child can reliably be determined.

FAMILY RELATIONSHIPS

It is often stated that IVF children are more desired than naturally conceived children. This clinical opinion was voiced since Louise Brown was born, and was more or less codified by a study of IVF children by Golombok[16]. Only one semi-rigorous study exists. In this study the views of Golombok appeared to be corroborated. Nevertheless, there is an important caveat to the study of Barnes *et al.*[17], namely, that although the study involved 1523 children and their families, response rates varied and thus representativeness has to be questioned; also, that the values in all the measures used to look at concerning these delicate relationships were normal *in all three* groups (IVF, ICSI, and natural conception). Thus, it was only the comparative that was different between the groups, not that the naturally conceived families were anything other than normal in their experiences as parents and in the experiences in relation to work, etc. More details of this and other studies can be seen in Chapter 6.

REFERENCES

1. Human Fertilisation and Embryology Authority. Seventh Annual Human Fertilisation and Embryology Authority Report. London: HFEA, 1998
2. Medical Research International Society for Assisted Reproductive Technology (SART) TAFS. In vitro fertilization–embryo transfer (IVF-ET) in the United States: 1990 results from IVF-ET Registry. Fertil Steril 1992; 5: 15–24
3. Cohen J, Mayaux MJ, Guihard-Moscato ML. Pregnancy outcomes after in vitro fertilization. A collaborative study on 2342 pregnancies. Ann NY Acad Sci 1988; 541: 1–6
4. Morin NC, Wirth FH, Johnson DH, et al. Congenital malformations and psychosocial development in children conceived by in vitro fertilization. J Pediatr 1989; 115: 222–7
5. Sharlip ID, Jarow JP, Belker AM, et al. Best practice policies for male infertility. Fertil Steril 2002; 77: 873–82
6. American Society for Reproductive Medicine/Society for Assisted Reproductive Technology. Assisted Reproductive Technology in the United States and Canada: 1995 results generated from the American Society for Reproductive Medicine/Society for Assisted Reproductive Technology Registry. Fertil Steril 1998; 69: 389–98
7. Yamamoto M, Watanabe G. Epidemiology of gross chromosomal anomalies at the early embryonic stage of pregnancy. Cont Epidemiol Biostat 1979; 1: 101–6
8. Office of Population Censuses and Surveys. London: HMSO, 1998
9. Angell RR. Aneuploidy in older women. Higher rates of aneuploidy in oocytes from older women. Hum Reprod 1994; 9: 1199–200

10. Smith KE, Buyalos RP. The profound impact of patient age on pregnancy outcome after early detection of fetal cardiac activity. Fertil Steril 1996; 65: 35–40

11. Hassold T, Abruzzo M, Adkins K, et al. Human aneuploidy: incidence, origin, and etiology. Environ Mol Mutagen 1996; 28: 167–75

12. Wyrobek AJ, Aardema M, Eichenlaub-Ritter U, et al. Mechanisms and targets involved in maternal and paternal age effects on numerical aneuploidy. Environ Mol Mutagen 1996; 28: 254–64

13. McIntosh GC, Olshan AF, Baird PA. Paternal age and the risk of birth defects in offspring. Epidemiology 1995; 6: 282–8

14. Yoshida A, Miura K, Shirai M. Cytogenetic survey of 1,007 infertile males. Urol Int 1997; 58: 166–76

15. Patrizio P, Asch RH, Handelin B, et al. Aetiology of congenital absence of vas deferens: genetic study of three generations. Hum Reprod 1993; 8: 215–20

16. Golombok S. Psychological functioning in infertility patients. Hum Reprod 1992; 7: 208–12

17. Barnes J, Sutcliffe AG, Kristoffersen I, et al. The influence of assisted reproduction on family functioning and children's socio-emotional development: results from a European study. Hum Reprod 2004; 19: 1480–7

Chapter 2

Methodological considerations when designing studies to examine the health of children born following ART

Jennifer J Kurinczuk, Michèle Hansen and Carol Bower

INTRODUCTION

The quality of the evidence produced by any scientific study is critically dependent on the study design. This chapter deals with issues that should be considered when designing studies to investigate the health outcomes of children born following assisted reproductive technology (ART) conception. The topics covered include identifying the research question(s); design issues including whether and when it is appropriate to use a 'matched' design and choosing appropriate comparison groups; data sources and data collection methods; sample size considerations; and analytical approaches. Examples from the literature have been included to illustrate particular points and are not intended to provide an exhaustive critique of all the studies that may be cited as examples of particular methodological points.

Published case series are often the starting point for further investigation of particular health problems and their association with ART, for example Angelman syndrome following intracytoplasmic sperm injection (ICSI)[1]. However, given the limited evidence that case series provide they will not be covered in this chapter.

THE RESEARCH QUESTION – WHAT DO YOU WANT TO FIND OUT?

Defining the research question(s) is the first fundamental step in any piece of research. The importance of how the research question is framed cannot be overemphasized. The entire design of the study that will follow hinges critically upon how the research question is framed, and then developed and elaborated into the study aims and objectives. The importance of this stage of the process should not be underestimated nor should it be rushed.

In assessing the health of children born following ART there is a wide range of health outcomes that are of interest. A list of potential areas to address, as described by Schieve et al.[2], is given in Table 2.1. The kind of questions that might be developed to examine these outcomes can be simplified into three main types.

Type I questions

The first type of research question relates to describing the incidence of an outcome following a particular exposure. For example, what is the incidence of twin delivery following in vitro fertilization (IVF) treatment? Or, what is the perinatal mortality rate following IVF treatment? The findings from this type of question can be used to counsel couples considering treatment about the likely chance (or risk) of a particular outcome, such as a twin birth or perinatal death. The results from this kind of question are

Table 2.1 Examples of outcomes of interest following conception by assisted reproductive technologies. Adapted from reference 2

Outcomes of interest	
Pregnancy	Infant morbidity
Multiple conception and birth	Birth defects in general
Spontaneous abortion	Specific birth defects and groups of defects
Late fetal loss	
Stillbirth	Imprinting-related disorders
Perinatal mortality	Childhood cancer
Perinatal morbidity	Developmental and cognitive outcomes
Low birth weight	Puberty-related disorders
Intrauterine growth restriction	Adult fertility
Preterm delivery	Many other rare and/or more subtle disorders
Infant mortality	

intended only to be descriptive and not comparative. Thus, the findings will be expressed as absolute outcome rates, for example, as described by Dhont *et al.*, a perinatal mortality rate of 13.5 per 1000 total births for ART singletons[3].

Type II questions

The second type of question, which effectively builds on the answers to the first type of question, is comparative. This type of question is therefore framed in comparative terms. For example: How does the incidence of a particular outcome (e.g. perinatal mortality) following ART compare with the incidence of perinatal mortality in another group, such as following spontaneous conception? The results from this type of question are intended to be comparative and, in addition to absolute outcome rates, will be expressed using comparative effect measures such as rate ratios, relative risks and odds ratios. An exploration of other risk factors and potential confounders is not required to answer this type of question and, as will be discussed later, inappropriate study design decisions, such as the decision to match the comparison population, may fatally flaw the ability of the study to provide the answer to this kind of primary comparative question.

Type III questions

The third type of research question, which builds upon findings from the first two questions, is also comparative, but in addition is intended to be explanatory. This kind of question will follow from the findings from a type II question such as the identification of a higher rate of perinatal mortality of singletons conceived following ART conception compared with spontaneous singletons[4,5]. The question will be framed in both a comparative and an explanatory form. For example: what factors might explain an excess risk of perinatal mortality experienced by women who have conceived following ART compared with women who conceived spontaneously?

As with type II questions, the comparative results will be expressed using comparative measures (rate ratio, relative risk, odds ratio), but a critical difference will be features of the study design that allow an exploration of the role of other risk factors and factors that may be confounders, such as maternal age, gestational age at delivery, birth weight and plurality. It is in anticipation of the exploration of the effects of confounding and how this might be conducted that critical study design decisions need to be made. The most crucial decision and one which cannot be undone in the analysis is whether or not to match the comparison group to the exposed group of interest with respect to potential confounding factors. Matching is an important method of confounder control, but it can have unintended consequences which are discussed later in the chapter along with other methods of dealing with the effects of confounding.

The decision about which type of research question it is desirable to answer at any particular point in time will depend on current knowledge in relation to the specific exposures and outcomes of interest. Clearly it is unlikely that an explanatory study to investigate the possible causes of an increased risk of perinatal mortality in singletons born following ART compared with spontaneous conception (type III question) would be embarked upon without prior knowledge of the rate of perinatal mortality following ART (type I question) or that the rate might be increased compared with spontaneous singletons (type II question).

The following sections outline aspects of study design, data collection and analysis, the approach to all of which may differ to some degree depending upon the extent of current knowledge and type of research question being addressed.

Defining the exposure of interest – which type of ART do you want to study?

The definition of the exposure or exposures of interest will follow from the research question. The more precisely the exposure can be defined the more specific the answer will be. It is often the case that different types of exposure are grouped together. This may be for several reasons including for convenience, to increase the study sample size or because the available data do not allow the separation of different groups. For example, in a study of congenital malformations in over 4000 children born following IVF, Anthony et al.[6] were unable to distinguish between IVF involving ICSI from IVF not involving ICSI, because the study was based on Dutch national register data which, at that time, did not make this distinction. Whilst this does not necessarily diminish the value of the results it clearly limited the capacity of the researchers to reach specific conclusions about anything other than the global effects of IVF. A clear definition of the exposure under investigation is crucial in both the conduct and the reporting of the study, the latter particularly so that other researchers understand the value and limitations of the findings.

Defining the outcome of interest – what health outcome are you interested in?

Again the outcome of interest will follow directly from the research question and the outcome must be clearly defined in measurable terms.

Difficulties arise when (1) there is no universally accepted definition for a particular outcome; (2) different data sources are used to assess the outcome for the exposed group and the comparison group; and (3) measures used to define the outcome for the exposed group are different from those used for the comparison group. Even when the same data sources and measures are used, (4) the outcome may not be adequately ascertained because the study design or the data source is inappropriate or incomplete; or (5) the outcome may be ascertained to a different extent for the different groups being compared.

The problem of the absence of a single, universally accepted definition of what constitutes a birth defect is a good example of the first and second difficulties. An early comparison of the rate of birth defects following ICSI conception used a narrow definition of what constitutes a major birth defect, but then the rate was compared to rates derived from data collected by birth defect registers or national data collections which used a much broader more inclusive definition of what constitutes a major birth defect[7]. The results suggested that there was no excess risk of birth defects following ICSI. Reclassification of the data and comparison with population-based data where both sets of data were classified using the same system to define the presence of a major birth defect suggested there was in fact an excess risk of major birth defects[8]; a finding which has subsequently been demonstrated in several further studies[9,10].

An example of the third problem occurred in a study by Verlaenen and colleagues[11] where children born following IVF were routinely examined by screening for the presence of birth defects, but the children in the spontaneously conceived comparison group were not. The additional screening consisted of an ultrasound examination of the heart and kidneys shortly after birth. Seven IVF infants were found to have (minor) heart malformations, five of which were detected by ultrasound and not at the physical examination. No malformations were found in the spontaneously conceived group who were not subject to the additional detailed examinations.

As regards the fourth problem, some studies have attempted to answer questions about outcomes which could not have been completely ascertained within the particular study design used. For example, in a study of developmental outcomes Sutcliffe et al.[12] identified a cohort of children conceived following frozen embryo transfer and compared their developmental attainment with a cohort of spontaneously conceived children of similar age, sex and social class; both cohorts were aged between 9 months and 3 years when examined. As an extension of the original study the investigators compared the prevalence of major and minor congenital anomalies and concluded that the rates were similar in both groups[13].

However, since children with malformations that have a high mortality around the time of birth or in infancy would not have survived to be included in the study, the results can be generalized only to infant survivors. Although the presence of birth defects in surviving children is clearly of interest, this study design could not address the fundamental issue of whether birth defects are more common overall following ART than spontaneous conception.

Finally, an example of a study in which the outcome may be ascertained to a different extent for both groups under comparison despite the same data source and measures being used is our own record linkage study assessing birth defects in children born following ART in Western Australia[14]. Birth defects were ascertained for both the ART and spontaneously conceived infants using the Western Australian Birth Defects Registry. However, it is possible that those obstetricians and pediatricians who knew of the conception method of ART infants more closely examined these children for the presence of birth defects. We attempted to address this issue by asking an independent pediatrician unaware of the conception status of the infants to exclude any defects that may have been identified because of closer surveillance and might not otherwise have been detected in a child less than 1 year of age; following which the excess risk was still evident.

THE STUDY DESIGN – HOW BEST TO CARRY OUT THE STUDY?

Choice of study design – cohort versus case–control study design

In order for something to be an outcome (for example multiple pregnancy) following from or associated with an exposure (for example ART) the exposure must, by definition, have preceded the outcome. In a study designed to identify the outcomes following ART the natural flow of evidence is therefore from the exposure to outcome. In this type of study, a group (or cohort) of individuals who have been exposed to the factor of interest (for example, conception by a specific ART procedure) are identified and followed forward over time to establish their status with regard to the outcome of interest. When the research question is a comparative one then an appropriate group (or cohort) of individuals who have not been exposed to the factor of interest are similarly identified and followed forward over time to establish their outcomes (Figure 2.1). The starting point of these types of studies is thus the exposure. Such studies are commonly referred to as cohort studies or longitudinal follow-up studies. In the

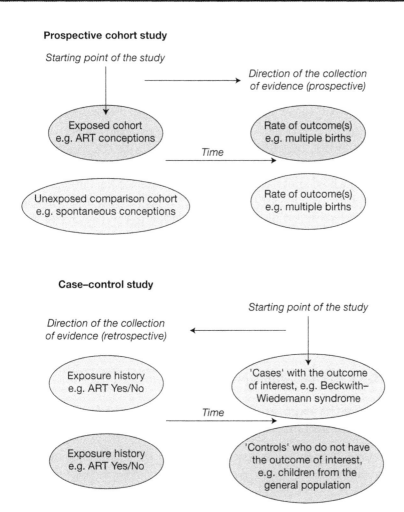

Figure 2.1 Schematic representation to compare the basic design features of a prospective cohort study and a case–control study

hierarchy of evidence used to establish causality the results from well-conducted cohort studies are regarded as second only to the results from randomized controlled trials in terms of the quality of the evidence they provide[15].

Most of this chapter will deal with the design and conduct of cohort studies in the investigation of outcomes following ART. There are, however, some circumstances when it is simply not possible to conduct a cohort study to answer a question about some specific outcome. This particularly arises when the outcome is so rare that the size of the cohorts (both exposed and unexposed) that would need to be followed forward to ensure that sufficient, or indeed any, children with the outcome are identified is prohibitively large. In these circumstances the study design required will be completely different and will start effectively at the end of the evidence trail by identifying children with the outcome of interest, for example Angelman syndrome, who are referred to as the 'cases'. The retrospectively ascertained exposure history (were they conceived following ART?) of the cases will then be compared with the exposure history (were they conceived following ART?) of an appropriately identified group of children who do not have the outcome of interest; the latter are referred to as 'controls'. Such 'case–control studies' come third after randomized controlled trials and cohort studies in relation to the strength of the evidence of causality they provide. This is mainly because they effectively start at the end with the outcome; do not follow the natural trail of the evidence; and data about exposure are usually collected retrospectively after the outcome is known, and hence are at greater risk of bias than the prospective collection of exposure data in cohort studies. The role of case–control studies is discussed briefly at the end of the chapter.

COHORT STUDY DESIGN

Identifying the exposed cohort of interest – which treatment group(s) are you interested in?

The source of both the exposed cohort and the comparison, unexposed cohort will be driven by the research question and will range from clinic-based cohorts, population-based cohorts assembled for special follow-up, to cohorts derived from IVF registers. Each approach has particular advantages and disadvantages and one may be more suitable for the investigation of particular research questions than the others.

Clinic-based cohorts

There are many examples in the literature of cohort studies of children born following ART treatment at a specific clinic. The advantages of this approach arise from the special relationship that often exists between successfully treated couples and their clinic. This usually leads to a high response to an invitation to participate in research and allows investigators access to clinic records. For example, 80% of the couples treated with IVF approached by Bowen et al.[16] at 28–30 weeks of pregnancy agreed to participate in a follow-up study of child development and 98% of the children of those women who originally agreed were subsequently assessed when they turned 1 year old. A further advantage of the clinic-based approach is that it may be possible to undertake more extensive data collection either by questionnaire to the parents or by examination of the children than might be the case in other circumstances, since the goodwill of parents may increase their tolerance. Thus, a protocol that requires a detailed clinical or psychological examination might be best approached via a clinic population. There are, however, several disadvantages to this approach.

On the whole, studies conducted using specific clinic patients tend to be small, although there are notable exceptions to this, for example the work of Bonduelle and colleagues[17]. The importance of appropriate study size and the limitations of studies that are too small and thus prone to false-negative findings are discussed in a later section of this chapter. The generalizability, that is the wider applicability, of the results may also be problematic, since a particular clinic may treat particular types of couples who have a specific range of problems. The bias that might arise in these circumstances is a form of 'selection bias' generally called 'referral bias'[18]. Results from a single clinic may therefore not be generally applicable to a wider group of couples seeking ART treatment. The impact of referral bias on the interpretation of the results and their wider applicability may be ameliorated by authors describing their study participants in detail.

While clinic-based studies may be able to achieve high participation rates, the potential problem of 'volunteer' or 'participation' bias (which is a form of selection bias) remains an issue in some of these studies. This type of bias arises when particular individuals eligible for inclusion in a study are more likely or less likely to agree to participate depending on their outcome status[18]. It may be the case that couples with children who have specific health problems are more likely or less likely to agree to participate in follow-up. If their child has a health problem the parents may be more likely to participate because they are interested in the research into health problems specifically because their child has a problem. Alternatively, they may be less likely to participate if their child has a serious disability. For example, their child's disability may make attending the follow-up appointment too difficult. Similarly, if their child is completely healthy the parents may misunderstand and believe that the researchers are only interested in children with health problems and therefore decline to participate. On the other hand, because their child is healthy access to the follow-up appointment may be easier and they may be more inclined to participate than if their child had a problem. The difficulty with volunteer bias is that, unless clinics have another source of information about the health status of the child they are following up, it is generally not possible to determine in which health status category those who do not agree to participate belong. Thus, it is not usually possible to assess to what extent bias is affecting the results. Nor is it usually possible to determine the direction of effect of the bias since, as illustrated above, the bias may lead to an underestimate or overestimate of health problems in either the ART cohort or the comparison cohort, depending upon who chooses to participate and the extent of non-participation.

Population-based cohorts assembled for special follow-up

In this particular type of study a cohort of ART children from a particular population is identified and invited to participate in follow-up. Such populations are usually defined by geography and time, rather than being simply from a single clinic. For example, researchers have assessed growth, psychomotor development and morbidity up to 3 years of age in all children born after IVF in Northern Finland 1990–1995. The children were identified by the only two IVF clinics serving the whole region[19].

The advantage of population-based cohort studies is that, when properly conducted, they avoid the problem of referral bias since they include all eligible children from a defined population. Also, in comparison with clinic-based studies, population-based studies tend to be larger, thus avoiding the problems of false-negative results associated with small samples. If such studies require patient contact and participation, they are, however, subject to the same potential problems of volunteer bias, as are clinic-based studies. Furthermore, as with clinic-based studies, if follow-up on more than one occasion is required, additional losses to follow-up may ensue.

A compromise in the extent of data collection may be necessary compared with clinic-based studies. For resource reasons it may not be possible to conduct a detailed examination of children when they number in the several hundreds, whereas, in clinic-based studies of fewer children it may be possible to carry out such examinations. The importance of this will depend on the research question being addressed; data collection issues are discussed in more detail in a later section.

Where high levels of participation are achieved, and thus volunteer bias minimized, population-based results are preferable to clinic-based findings, as the results will be more widely applicable.

Register-based cohort studies

The problems of volunteer bias which may arise in both clinic-based and population-based follow-up studies may be avoided by using IVF registers as the source of the study cohort. When statutory population-based IVF registers, such as those in Denmark and Western Australia, are used, the issue of the failure to identify and include all eligible children is avoided. Linkage of IVF registers to other registers of health outcomes generally avoids completely the problem of volunteer (thus selection) bias and bias resulting from losses to follow-up. Register-based studies with data collected over a number of years in a reasonably sized population also have the advantage of large sample size. For example, the register-based cohort of Danish ART infants now includes close to 20 000 infants (A Pinborg, personal communication).The limited financial cost associated with using data that have already been collected is a further advantage compared with studies that require the collection of data specifically for a study. Register-based studies have been used to investigate the relationship between ART and the risk of birth defects by linking IVF data to birth defects register data. Other outcomes investigated in this way to date include stillbirth, preterm birth, low birth weight, neonatal death, admission to hospital, visual impairment and childhood cancer.

Register-based studies in jurisdictions that do not require contact with participants avoid completely the problems of volunteer (thus selection) bias and bias resulting from losses to follow-up, since participants are not asked whether they wish to participate in the study. These studies usually involve record linkage of ART registers to other population-based health registers and incorporate strict confidentiality requirements such that the data once linked are analyzed anonymously and the results cannot be used in any way to identify individual participants.

As with other types of study design register-based studies also have some limitations. The first relates to access to the information for research purposes. Whilst some jurisdictions collect IVF information under statute and thus reliably identify all eligible children, access to that information for research purposes may be limited. For example, the data collected by the Human Fertilisation and Embryology Authority in the UK have not been linked to health outcome data. Second, in circumstances where non-statutory register data that identify IVF children are available for research purposes it is wise to check that they do indeed cover the entire eligible population of children. For example, the children born following IVF in Finland are identified using information collected from mothers at delivery and recorded on the birth register. The register custodians have estimated that at least 15% of eligible children are not identified using this method[20].

Third, there may be limitations in the extent of the data collected on the IVF register. The information may not include sufficient detail about the exposure of interest; for example, some ART data collections cannot distinguish between IVF and ICSI treatment and there are currently no national ART data collections that incorporate information about non-IVF ovulation induction treatment. Information about potential confounding factors may be missing; for example, there may be only limited paternal information. Finally, although an ART register may be available it may not include identifying information necessary for record linkage to population-based health registers in order to assess health outcomes of interest. This is the case in many countries such as Germany, France and the USA. Register-based cohort studies work best in places that allow record linkage to many different population-based health outcome registers as, for example, in Denmark, Sweden and Western Australia.

Identifying an appropriate 'unexposed' comparison group – with whom do you wish to make a comparison?

As with the choice of ART cohort, the choice of an appropriate comparison group is driven by the research question. Again, as in the case of the exposed cohort, there are several sources from which comparison group information can be obtained.

Comparison group not required

If the purpose of the research is to answer a type I research question and describe the incidence of a particular health outcome, for example perinatal mortality, without any comparative intention then self-evidently a comparison cohort will not be required.

Routinely available information

In the case of a comparative, type II, research question where the comparison is with the general population of births, infants or children, there are some health outcomes for which routinely collected information is available from statutory sources. For example, in the UK the Office for National Statistics routinely publishes perinatal mortality rates for the population of England and Wales and the Information and Statistics Division of the Scottish Health Service publishes the Scottish rates. The main limitation of routinely available statistics is that in most places they are available for relatively few health-related outcomes. The quality of routinely collected data may also vary. Statutorily collected data, such as mortality statistics, generally represent the highest quality data. The quality of other data collections (non-statutory and statutory) should be checked before comparisons are made[21]. An important aspect of using these data for comparison purposes is that the outcome in both the exposed and comparison groups should be collected using the same definition, over the same time period, and be equally well ascertained in both groups, otherwise bias may creep into the comparison. The more clearly defined, unambiguous and well ascertained the outcome, the less prone to bias the comparison will be.

Population-based cohorts assembled for special follow-up

When the research question is a type III comparative question and the researchers wish to explore in more detail the relationship between exposure to a particular treatment and the health outcome of interest, more information will usually be required than can be provided by most routinely available statistics. In this situation when the cohort of children born following ART is identified (exposed group) and invited to participate in the study, ideally the investigators would simultaneously identify a suitable comparison group. Thus, participation and follow-up of both groups would occur at the same time.

Which particular group of children would best constitute a suitable comparator will depend upon the research question being investigated. For example, there has been much debate recently about whether increased risks of birth defects in children born following ART may be attributable to some aspect of the ART treatment or to the underlying infertility of the couple seeking treatment. In order to answer this question it would be helpful to compare the prevalence of birth defects in the children born to couples in a number of different groups: (1) infertile couples who have had IVF; (2) originally fertile couples now sterile through vasectomy or tubal ligation who required IVF to conceive; (3) infertile couples who have had non-IVF ART such as ovulation induction with oral clomiphene citrate; (4) infertile couples who have not had any form of ART but after a prolonged period conceive spontaneously; and (5) fertile couples who have not had ART (spontaneous conceptions). It is clear from this list that the term 'unexposed' comparison cohort is a relative one which, depending upon the research question, can be taken to mean not exposed to IVF but exposed to other forms of infertility treatment.

The source of the comparison cohort will be very different depending upon which of the groups listed above is chosen for comparison. Assuming that the first group (infertile couples who had IVF) is the exposed group of interest and the second group (iatrogenically sterile couples who required IVF to conceive) have been identified as the appropriate group for comparison, it is clear that both groups would have to be recruited through IVF clinics although on a population basis to avoid the problems of clinic-based studies or, if the appropriate data are available, identified in IVF register data. In this situation both groups would be relatively easy to identify.

It will be more difficult to identify suitable participants if the third group (infertile couples treated with non-IVF ART) was deemed the most appropriate comparator. Whilst some of these couples will be treated in infertility clinics, in many places treatment such as clomiphene citrate is prescribed by non-specialists in other settings, for example general gynecology clinics or general practice. Whilst it might be possible to recruit on a population basis those women attending infertility clinics, caution would be required, as it is possible that those couples treated by specialist clinics might differ in important ways from those couples not referred for specialist infertility advice. Such differences risk introducing bias into any comparison.

The fourth group (prolonged time to conception but conceived without requiring ART) is probably the most difficult group to identify in sufficient numbers and in an unbiased way, since they may never come to the attention of infertility specialists or general gynecologists. In contrast to the first three groups, the fourth and fifth groups will have to be identified from the general population of births and the conception history ascertained at that stage. An alternative approach, in well-funded circumstances, is to recruit a group of women who are planning a pregnancy and follow them forward in time[22]. Provided that the cohort is sufficiently large, several groups will eventually self-identify as their attempts to conceive succeed or fail. These will include women who conceive rapidly or at least within a defined period of time such as 1 or 2 years; women who eventually conceive spontaneously, after a defined period, such as 1 or 2 years (prolonged time to conception); women who conceive following non-IVF infertility treatment; women who require IVF to conceive; women who do not conceive and choose not to pursue treatment; women who have infertility treatment but without success; and women who change their mind about wishing to become pregnant and do not continue to try to conceive. Furthermore, some women initially enrolled in follow-up will, for a variety of reasons, be lost to follow-up and it will not be possible to identify into which outcome group they fall.

One of the major limiting factors of this approach is the fortunate reality that the number of women requiring and seeking infertility treatment in population terms is relatively small. The initial cohort that would need to be recruited in order to result in informative numbers of ART births will be very large[22]. Follow-up on this scale also takes a long time. As a consequence of these two factors this type of follow-up study is very costly since not only will it be necessary to follow the women to conception but, depending upon the child health outcome of interest, it may be necessary to continue follow-up of those who successfully deliver for a long period of time after their baby is born. The follow-up process is also rather more complicated than this very simplistic linear description implies since, over time, women may move from group to group. This is particularly true for women who have difficulty conceiving as they may choose to pursue different treatment options at different points in time but then change their mind about wishing to conceive at all.

The major advantage of this approach is that the outcomes associated with a whole range of different fertility and treatment experiences can be compared, thus enabling both comparative and exploratory analyses to be performed to answer many research questions.

Special case: the 'matched' comparison cohort

Having identified a suitable source or sampling frame from which a comparison cohort of pregnancies or children can be drawn, the next question is whether the comparison cohort should be drawn as a random sample or as a 'matched' or 'restricted' sample. Matching in this situation refers to the selection of specific individuals from the comparison pregnancies/children with characteristics that are the same (or very similar) to the characteristics of the individual pregnancies/children in the exposed cohort. Whether or not it is appropriate to carry out matching depends entirely on the research question that is being addressed. The sole purpose of matching is to deal with the effects of confounding and hence the characteristics upon which subjects are matched must be known or potential confounders for the research question of interest. Matching is not the only method that can be used for dealing with the effects of confounding. However, since matching is implemented during the course of a study, a decision about whether or not to match has to be made in the design stage.

Once the decision to match has been made and implemented, the effects of matching are irrevocable and cannot be 'undone' in the analysis. For this reason it is strongly recommended that investigators think very carefully in the design stage about whether matching is the appropriate strategy to control confounding and consider the alternative approaches before making a final decision.

Matching should only be considered when researchers are attempting to answer a type III comparative research question. That is, when it is known that there is an excess rate of a particular outcome in the ART group compared to spontaneously conceived singleton pregnancies, for example, perinatal mortality, and the investigation of the issue has now moved on to the stage of trying to understand and explain why this might be so.

Matching is a method to deal in the study design with the effects of confounding factors. A confounder is a factor that is both independently associated with the exposure of interest *and* is causally related to or predictive of the outcome of interest (Figure 2.2)[23]. In the situation of ART the exposure of interest is infertility treatment (or not), for example IVF, and the outcome is the specific health outcome of interest, for example birth defects. An example of a factor that may be a confounder in this particular situation is maternal age (Figure 2.3). Maternal age is a potential confounder since there is an association between higher maternal age and the need for IVF and independently of this there is also an association between maternal age and the risk of some birth defects, specifically chromosomal anomalies. Whilst maternal age may be regarded as a potential confounder, whether or not it actually is a confounder in any particular situation can only be demonstrated by examining this in the analysis. For example, in this case one would look for evidence of a relationship between maternal age and receipt of IVF *and* for a relationship between maternal age and the risk of birth defects. If a relationship exists between maternal age and only one of the factors, i.e. receipt of IVF or risk of birth defects, and not between both, then maternal age in this situation is not actually a confounder, although this may not be the case in other studies.

Matching assumes that all the potential confounding factors matched in the design are in reality actual confounders. Furthermore, once these

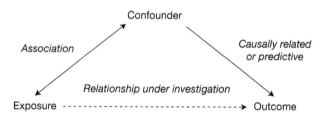

Figure 2.2 Schematic representation of the relationship between an exposure, outcome and a confounding variable

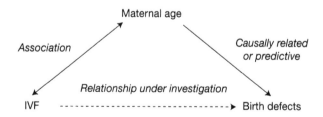

Figure 2.3 Example of maternal age as a confounder in the relationship between exposure to IVF and birth defects as the outcome

factors have been matched in the study it is not possible to test whether in fact a confounding relationship exists; it remains assumed. For factors that are real confounders close matching provides a powerful method for dealing with, that is removing, their effects from the study results. By making the comparison (e.g. spontaneous conceptions) cohort the same (or very similar) to the exposed cohort (e.g. IVF conceptions) with respect to a potential confounder (e.g. maternal age) then any differences between the two groups in terms of the risk of the outcome (e.g. perinatal death) cannot be explained by the effects of the confounding factor that has been matched (e.g. maternal age). This does not, however, necessarily confirm that maternal age was a confounder, it simply means that any excess risk demonstrated is not due to the effects of maternal age. Furthermore, by matching it is not now possible to examine the relationship between the risk of the outcome and maternal age.

The second advantage of close matching is that once carried out the investigators need not concern themselves with the effects of the matched factor any further. The third advantage of matching is that it is statistically efficient, that is fewer individuals in both cohorts will be required to achieve the same study power compared with an unmatched design. Fourth, matching is often a practical approach to selecting the comparison cohort. That is when individuals in the exposed cohort are identified and approached there are often practical advantages to identifying and approaching the unexposed comparison individuals at the same time. Finally, it is sometimes possible to match on one factor that can lead to adjustment for the confounding effects of a wide range of factors. This can be desirable in some circumstances for a variable such as neighbourhood or school peers, as it will lead to adjustment for a wide range of social and economic factors that would otherwise be difficult, if not impossible, to identify and measure[24]. Care must be taken, however, as it is also possible that this type of matching leads to inadvertent over-matching with unanticipated and undesirable consequences.

The major disadvantage of matching, as noted above, is that once matching has been carried out it cannot be undone and it will not be possible for the investigators to examine at a later stage the relationship between the exposure and the matched characteristic or the outcome and the matched characteristic.

In addition to the inability to 'undo' the effects of matching, there are several other disadvantages. One is that it is possible to match on characteristics that are not only *not* confounders but are in fact factors on the causal pathway between the exposure and the outcome. By this we mean factors that have a relationship with both the exposure and the outcome but that relationship is not an independent one and the factor is part of the chain of events that leads from the exposure to the outcome. Matching on causal factors is one form of so-called 'over-matching' and its effects will be to mask the real risk relationship between the exposure and the outcome. Another disadvantage is that some investigators attempt to match on so many characteristics that they are unable to find matches in the comparison group for all the individuals in the exposed group. This often leads them to discard the data of individuals without matches from the analysis, which is wasteful in terms of both resources and the power of the study. This occurred in the study of the obstetric outcomes of twin pregnancies after IVF where Koudstaal et al.[25] attempted to match the IVF twin pregnancies to spontaneous twins on seven separate characteristics. They were only able to find suitable matches for 96 of the original 144 twin pregnancies eligible for inclusion; thus excluding 33% of their potential study subjects on this basis.

A further disadvantage is that, whilst matching may be a statistically efficient approach, it is not necessarily efficient in terms of cost. If a cohort is being assembled for special follow-up it is usually necessary to conduct some sort of screening process to identify individuals as appropriate matches and this can be costly. Whatever method is used to identify matches, if the matching is not 'close', i.e. the individuals are not sufficiently similar, the effects of confounding will not have been completely dealt with, leading to the disadvantage of so-called 'residual confounding'. Whilst residual confounding can be dealt with in the analysis (see below) researchers in the IVF field rarely appear to consider this option.

Care must also be taken when matching to ensure that, by matching on one factor, other factors are not inadvertently and undesirably matched. For example, in studies of perinatal outcome, unexposed cohort matches are commonly identified from the same place of delivery as the exposed cohort[26]. The potential problem with matching on this seemingly innocuous variable is that it may inadvertently lead to matching on the outcome of interest. This is likely to happen because IVF pregnancies are more likely to be delivered in a tertiary obstetric unit than spontaneous pregnancies and, independently of this, adverse outcomes are more likely to occur in spontaneous pregnancies referred to such high-risk units for management and delivery. Matching on place of delivery is therefore likely to lead to an over-representation of adverse outcomes in the comparison cohort than if randomly selected pregnancies had been included. Such an over-matched comparison will lead to an underestimate of the comparative rate of adverse outcomes[27].

Finally, many investigators appear to assume that matching is automatically the best approach to confounder control without considering the alternatives of dealing with the effects of confounders in the analysis by either stratification methods (for a small number of factors) or regression methods to carry out adjusted analyses (see the analysis section below for a more complete discussion of these options).

COLLECTING THE OUTCOME DATA – HOW BEST TO COLLECT THE INFORMATION NEEDED?

The sources of data and methods of data collection are crucial to the validity of the research findings of any study. There are three main methods of ascertaining health outcomes for children born following ART and the choice of a particular method will depend upon the research question, the rarity of the outcomes, logistical and resource considerations. The first method involves patient participation in the form of completion of a postal questionnaire by the parents, an interview with the parents and/or child, or some sort of medical examination or assessment of the children. The second method involves a search of medical records for study children. For example, in a study of growth, psychomotor development and morbidity up to 3 years of age in children born after IVF in Northern Finland, researchers manually searched child health center records and hospital notes to collect health outcome information for all study participants[19]. The third method of ascertaining health outcomes in children born following ART involves record linkage to a data source that identifies the outcome of interest. Register-based studies have been used to investigate the relationship between ART and the risk of adverse neonatal outcomes (such as stillbirth, preterm birth, low birth weight and neonatal death) by linking IVF data to registers of birth, for example the study by Pinborg *et al.*[28].

Of particular importance in the types of study discussed here is the need to collect information using the same methods and in the same way for all groups being followed up, thus avoiding or at least minimizing the chance of 'information bias'. Information bias arises when the data collection occurs differentially between the groups, leading to better, more complete information in one group compared with the other[18]. This can arise because one group is, for example, more closely examined than the other group, or if one group reports outcomes in more detail. An example of the latter would be if parents of children born after ART provided more (or less) detail than the parents of comparison children in response to a questionnaire about their child's health.

Ideally data should be collected from sources of information that provide an objective measure of the variables of interest. Subjective data are best avoided unless it is the specific focus of the research, in which case pre-validated data collection instruments should be used. Good-quality outcome information collected without knowledge of exposure status (i.e. without knowing from which conception group the children come) is preferable. Such 'blinding' to the exposure status may be possible to achieve relatively easily if the data about both exposure and outcome are collected from already documented sources. If, however, the parents and children themselves are involved in providing the data or in undergoing specific examinations it may not be possible to keep the interviewer or examiner 'blind' to conception exposure status. The lack of blinding leads to the risk of what is generally known as 'interviewer bias' or 'observer bias' which is a particular form of 'information bias'[18]. The bias arises in this situation because the interviewer or examiner potentially treats one of the groups differently to the other group either consciously or more probably unconsciously; that is, they question or examine one group more thoroughly or less thoroughly than the other.

In most cohort studies, exposure information is recorded before the outcomes of interest are known and so cannot be subject to 'information bias' since the outcome was not known when the exposure information was collected. However, to avoid completely the risk of introducing information bias the outcome information must also then be collected without knowledge of exposure status, or the outcome itself must be a 'hard' outcome that cannot be subject to differential ascertainment between the groups. For example, ascertainment of perinatal death is unlikely to be subject to bias unless a very unreliable source of information is used to identify deaths in one cohort and a highly reliable source is used for the other cohort.

Limitations associated with ascertaining health outcomes through register-based record linkage studies include the fact that some conditions such as development and cognitive milestones are rarely collected in routine statistics or disease registers and therefore cannot be assessed in this way. In addition, although a particular register (such as a register of births) may include information about the outcome of interest to the study (e.g. birth defects) this condition may not be adequately ascertained by the register. It is known, for example, that about one-third of birth defects are not clinically obvious at birth and may not be diagnosed at this time, so that assessment of birth defects by record linkage with a birth register may underestimate the prevalence of birth defects (in both the exposed and the unexposed children) compared with record linkage to a high-quality birth defects register which collects information about defects diagnosed up to later ages.

The design of the data collection instrument, whether it is used to collect information from a documentary source, interview or examination, is critical to the production of valid results. The instrument should be designed prior to the data collection stage and ideally piloted on a sample of both the exposed and the unexposed cohorts to ensure that the data are feasible to collect and that the instrument is collecting the information that will be needed to answer the research question posed. One common mistake is to omit data items relating to important potential confounding factors. Whilst it might be a self-evident fact that the effects of confounders can be dealt with in the analysis only if data about them are collected, failure to collect information about important confounders is not an uncommon error.

Data should also preferably be collected in as 'raw' a form as possible. That is, it is preferable to collect, for example maternal age in years or mother's date of birth, rather than in pre-determined groups (< 20 years, 20–24 years, 25–29 years and so on). Whilst the investigator may have pre-specified groups in mind to use in the analysis, raw unit data allow the groups to be altered, whereas data collected in pre-specified groups cannot be ungrouped. This is of particular importance in relation to confounding factors, since adjusting for confounders using pre-grouped data can be subject to incomplete adjustment if the distribution of maternal age even within relatively narrow groups is different between the exposed and the unexposed cohorts. This incomplete adjustment can lead to residual confounding.

SAMPLE SIZE AND STUDY POWER – HOW BIG SHOULD THE STUDY BE?

The size of a study has a major impact on the precision of the study's findings. In the way that we would not allow the outcome of a general election to be based on the voting preferences of ten electors, we would not be very convinced by the results of a study based on so few subjects. The two main questions in research study design in relation to the size of the study are: how big is big enough, and can we ever reach the point of including too many research subjects? The inclusion of too many subjects wastes resources that could be better spent answering other important research questions. The inclusion of too few subjects risks failing to identify as statistically significant an increased or decreased risk associated with a particular exposure when in reality such an increase or decrease actually exists, i.e. a false-negative finding.

The power of a study is the ability of the study to detect as statistically significant an effect, i.e. an increased or a decreased risk, which in reality exists; power is the complement of the chance of missing a real effect[18]. For example, if a study is so small that it only has 50% power this means there is only a 50:50 chance of detecting as statistically significant an increase in relative risk associated with a particular exposure when in reality this increased risk exists. This is equivalent to tossing a coin to determine the result. Conventionally acceptable levels of power start at 80%, although 90%, 95%, or even 99% power is preferable but rarely achievable, owing to resource limitations in many settings.

The derivation of sample sizes is a process of estimation based on a series of generally well-informed guesses and decisions. The information needed to inform and thus estimate the sample size for a cohort study is as follows: (1) an estimate of the prevalence of the outcome of interest in the unexposed comparison group (e.g. perinatal mortality rate in spontaneously conceived infants); (2) a decision about the size of effect that is clinically important to be able to detect (e.g. a relative risk of two or more); (3) a decision about the acceptable level of power which is usually as a minimum 80% but preferably 90% or 95%; (4) a decision about the ratio of exposed to comparison subjects in the study, as it is usual to have either equal numbers of exposed and unexposed or a greater number of unexposed than exposed, simply because it is usually more difficult to increase the numbers in the exposed group than the comparison group; and (5) a decision about the acceptable level of statistical significance that will result from a two-sided significance test which is conventionally set at $p < 0.05$ but may be more stringently set at $p < 0.01$ or less stringently set at $p < 0.10$ if the study is exploratory.

It is commonly believed that if there is a fixed number of research subjects in one cohort (which is generally the exposed cohort) and hence the maximum number of subjects has been included, then a sample size or power calculation is not necessary. This, however, is far from the case. First it is important to calculate the study power, since this gives an indication of whether, if the study goes ahead, it will have sufficient power to detect a clinically important effect or whether it would have such low power (e.g. 50% or less) that the research resources would be better directed elsewhere. Second, although it may not be possible to increase the size of one of the groups (usually the exposed cohort) it may be possible to recruit a greater number in the comparison group, which will increase the power; five comparison subjects per exposed subject is the maximum recommended, as after that resource implications are outweighed by the very marginal increase in power[23]. It may also be possible to increase the study size and thus power by recruiting study subjects for longer than originally planned.

Studies need to be surprisingly large, mainly because adverse outcomes tend, fortunately, to be relatively uncommon. For example, to have an 80% chance (power) of detecting a doubling in the risk, at the 5% level of statistical significance, of an outcome in a group of ART children that occurs in the comparison population with a prevalence of 2%, a study would require a minimum of 724 ART children and 3620 (five times as many) children in the comparison cohort[29]. To detect smaller yet still clinically significant increases in risk for the same outcome would require larger numbers of children in both groups. Similarly, adverse outcomes that occur at a lower prevalence would also require a larger sample size. Table 2.2 gives an indication of the sample sizes required to detect a range of relative risks for a range of prevalence estimates[29]. This table was originally constructed to demonstrate the sample sizes required for studies of birth defects, but the figures can be applied to any outcome that occurs in the comparison cohort with a prevalence or cumulative incidence of 1% to 8%.

Doyle and colleagues estimated the sample size requirements for studies of childhood cancer following ART and demonstrated that for this very rare outcome (childhood cancer overall) 20 000 ART children followed for 5 years would be required[30]. Obviously, to look at specific cancers would require an even larger cohort.

Evidence of an a priori sample size calculation is rarely seen in publications of follow-up studies of ART children. This may be because authors or editors think that readers would not be interested in this information. Alternatively, it may be because investigators do not include such calculations in their study planning. As part of a recent review of comparative

Table 2.2 Estimated number of children exposed to ART required to investigate the risk of an outcome which occurs with a frequency between 1% and 8% in the comparison cohort, for a range of relative risks between 1.2 and 2.0, assuming that the unmatched comparison cohort includes five children for every child conceived by ART, with 80% power at the 5% level of statistical significance. Adapted from reference 29

Prevalence (%) of the outcome in the comparison cohort	Number of children exposed to ART required:		
	to detect a relative risk of 1.2	to detect a relative risk of 1.5	to detect a relative risk of 2.0
1	26 176	4752	1491
2	12 654	2414	724
4	6 797	1246	378
6	4 650	858	262
8	3 581	665	205

studies looking at the risk of birth defects in children born following ART we found that only five of the 26 studies eligible for inclusion were of sufficient size to detect as statistically significant a relative risk of 1.5 and only one was large enough to detect a smaller, but still clinically important, relative risk of 1.2[29].

ANALYSIS AND INTERPRETATION – WHAT DOES IT ALL MEAN?

Since this chapter is not intended to provide a comprehensive approach to the statistical analysis of cohort data we have confined ourselves to discussing four important issues. The first issue relates to analyses that depend solely for their interpretation on statistical significance testing. The second is the use of comparative effect measures (e.g. relative risk estimates) and 95% confidence intervals. The third relates to absolute versus relative effect measures. The final issue is that of dealing with the effects of confounding.

The purpose of statistical significance testing within the framework of hypothesis testing is to provide an indication of the role that chance may play in the study results. It is conventionally accepted that with $p < 0.05$ (i.e. chance is likely to account for the result observed in only 5 out of 100 (1 in 20) instances) chance is an unlikely explanation of the findings. Conversely, it is accepted that with $p > 0.05$ chance remains a possible explanation for the results observed; the role of chance cannot be excluded. It should be noted, however, that with $p > 0.05$ this is not the same as saying that chance is the cause of the result, nor is this the same as saying there is no difference between the groups: both common and mistaken interpretations. The results of significance testing give no indication of the size or direction of any differences between the groups being compared; they simply tell us about the role that chance may have played in their genesis.

Despite great encouragement to the contrary, many investigators still rely solely on the results of statistical significance testing in the comparison and interpretation of the outcomes of two or more groups[31]. The problem of relying solely on the interpretation of significance testing particularly relates to small studies which from the outset include insufficient subjects to detect even quite large differences between groups. For example, in 1989 in one of the first studies to examine the rate of birth defects in children born following ART, Morin and colleagues compared the rate of birth defects in 83 IVF children conceived following treatment in their clinic with 93 randomly selected children born in the local area[32]. Only two (2.4%) infants conceived by IVF had a major congenital anomaly, as did only one (1.1%) of the comparison cohort. On the basis of a statistical significance test (exact McNemar test, $p = 0.50$) the authors concluded that this difference was not statistically significant and concluded from this that 'no association between IVF and an increased risk of congenital malformations could be found'[32]. The authors were quite right to conclude that the result was not statistically significant and that the role of chance in producing the difference of 2.4% versus 1.1% could not be excluded. The difficulty arose in what they inferred from this, namely that this result demonstrated no association between the exposure and the outcome. In fact, this study was quite simply not large enough to reach this conclusion and had only 3% power to detect as statistically significant a relative risk of 2.2.

The combination of lack of power, relying solely on statistical significance testing and inappropriate interpretation of the results of significance testing led Morin and colleagues to fail to notice that in reality their data were showing evidence of over a two-fold increase in the relative risk of major birth defects (odds ratio 2.27). Of course, because the result was based on so few observations, the 95% confidence interval (which the authors did not calculate) around the relative risk estimate was very wide, at 0.20 to 25.5. A more appropriate interpretation of the results would be to say that the point estimate result (2.27) suggests there is over a two-fold increase in the risk of major birth defects, that the role of chance cannot be excluded and that the results are consistent with an 80% decrease in the risk of birth defects (lower bound of confidence interval 0.2) and up to a 25-fold increase (upper bound of confidence interval 25.5). A true elevated risk cannot be excluded by these data – this would require larger studies to be undertaken. In fact on the basis of these results there is a 75% probability that the true relative risk is greater than one[29]. Table 2.2 shows just how far the sample size in this study was adrift from the numbers needed to demonstrate a statistically significant result of this magnitude (relative risk 2.0) when the comparison cohort experienced the outcome at a prevalence of about 1%: 1491 needed in the ART group compared with 7455 in the comparison group.

The example given above demonstrates how much extra information an effect measure, in this case either a relative risk or an odds ratio, and its 95% confidence interval gives to the interpretation of study findings. Both absolute and relative effect measures are important from the point of view of understanding the etiology of the outcome. However, effect measures must be placed into perspective since if they are presented alone without the context of the absolute risk they can lead to alarm. For example, a doubling in the relative effect measure (relative risk 2.0) of birth defects in ART infants is of considerable concern and raises questions about what the causes might be. In a population where 4.2% of births have a birth defect, this means that 9% of ART infants have a birth defect (absolute effect measure)[14]. Whilst some couples may view this as alarming, it also means that 91% of ART infants will not have a birth defect – perhaps a more reassuring figure for some couples contemplating ART.

The final issue for discussion in this section relates to dealing with the effects of confounders. The use of matching techniques as one method for dealing with confounding has already been discussed. We suggest that matching should not be used for vast numbers of variables, since it becomes difficult if not impossible to find sufficient matches and, if the matching is not sufficiently close, some effects of the confounding may remain; this is called residual confounding. Two alternative methods of dealing with confounding are stratification and regression techniques. Stratification is the simplest of these and is commonly used in the analysis of ART data. For example, the results for singletons are quite often sepa-rated from the results relating to twins. Once the two groups are stratified in this way it is self-evident that the results from singletons cannot be influenced by results from the twins and vice versa. Thus, by stratifying by plurality the confounding effects of plural birth have been eliminated from the results relating to each stratum, i.e. we have dealt with the effects of plural birth as a confounder. It is possible, if the dataset is large enough, to stratify for more than one common variable at a time. However, as soon as stratification is attempted simultaneously for more than two variables, an extremely large dataset is required to ensure that many cells in the various strata are not empty, since the analysis breaks down when empty cells are produced. Thus, simple stratification is very useful but has its limitations as the sole means of confounder control.

Stratification is very useful and can be used in combination with the statistical regression techniques to adjust for several potential confounders simultaneously. For example, following stratification by plurality, other confounders can be adjusted for by using multivariate regression methods. Logistic and other forms of regression are now computationally simple when performed in commonly available statistical software such as SPSS, SAS and STATA. Their deceptive simplicity can, however, lead to the indiscriminate adjustment for factors that are either not confounders or are factors on the causal pathway between the exposure and the outcome. It is also important to test the statistical 'fit' of the models created using these types of analytical method and to consider their biological basis and meaning.

As noted above, residual confounding can result when the matching of two variables is not sufficiently close, for example maternal age matching that results in a difference in average age remaining between the two groups. This can subsequently be adjusted for in the analysis stage using regression techniques, thus eliminating the residual effects of the confounder. To avoid the problem of failing to find matches for all the exposed group it is suggested that matching, if used at all, is used for only a small number of key confounders and that remaining variables and any residual confounding is dealt with by regression techniques in the analysis[24].

THE ROLE OF CASE–CONTROL STUDIES

As discussed earlier, case–control studies are not follow-up studies and as such are not the focus of this chapter. We mention them here briefly because they can have an important role to play in the investigation between exposure to ART and specific outcomes in the framework of 'type III' research questions. The methodological strengths of case–control studies lie in their use to investigate the relationship between a range of potential exposures and a single rare outcome. Case–control studies are particularly useful when an outcome is so rare that it would require a prohibitively large cohort of ART-exposed pregnancies to be followed to identify sufficient numbers of children with the outcome for a meaningful analysis to be conducted. Rare outcomes can be investigated in a cohort methodology using record linkage methods if they are collected systematically in disease registers covering a defined population. For example, the relationship between ART and childhood cancers has been investigated this way, although the sample size remains an issue in this instance[33]. If, however, children with the rare outcome of interest are not included in a disease register, then a properly conducted case–control study may provide an alternative investigative route.

As illustrated in Figure 2.1, case–control studies take as their starting point a group of children with the outcome of interest; these are the 'cases'. A group of children is then identified who do not have the outcome and they act as the 'controls'. Thus, case–control studies start at the end of the natural trail of evidence between exposure and outcome. The history of exposure to the factor of interest (ART in this situation) and other factors of interest (including potential confounders) is collected for both cases and controls, either by interview or preferably from prerecorded documentary sources. The latter is preferable as it reduces the risk of one important sort of bias to which case–control studies tend to be susceptible, namely a form of information bias called 'recall' bias. Recall bias arises because of differential recall, questioning or recording of information between the cases and controls[18].

Provided that the cases are selected without reference to their exposure history and thus selection bias is avoided, and controls are similarly recruited without reference to their exposure history, and the exposure history is collected in an unbiased fashion, then the results from case–control studies can provide important evidence of the presence or absence of a relationship between the exposure(s) and outcome of interest in the form of a relative effect measure (an odds ratio). There is one other important difference between case–control studies and cohort studies which is that, unless the investigator is in the unusual situation of knowing that they have identified all eligible cases in a specified population for which the appropriate denominator is known, it is not usually possible to estimate absolute effect measures, i.e. incidence rates.

An example of the value of a case–control study is in investigating the suggestion of an increased risk of imprinting disorders such as Angelman syndrome and Beckwith–Wiedemann syndrome in infants born following ART. Given the rarity of these conditions in the general population (1/300 000 births for Angelman syndrome and 1/15 000 births for Beckwith–Wiedemann syndrome), case–control studies provide a more appropriate means than cohort studies of assessing any association with ART treatment. Halliday and colleagues[34] have carried out a case–control study examining ART exposure in Beckwith–Wiedemann syndrome cases and controls without Beckwith–Wiedemann syndrome in an Australian population and, because they were able to identify all eligible cases of Beckwith–Wiedemann syndrome in their population and also had population data on all births and all ART births, they were also able to estimate an absolute effect measure[34]. Thirty-seven cases of Beckwith–Wiedemann syndrome were identified among ~1 316 500 live births in Victoria between 1983 and 2003, giving an overall prevalence of ~1/35 580 live births for this period. For each Beckwith–Wiedemann syndrome case, four liveborn controls were selected from the State Birth Register (matched on maternal age and date of birth within 1 month of the case). IVF was found to be the method of conception in four Beckwith–Wiedemann syndrome cases and in one control, giving an odds ratio estimate of 17.8 (95% confidence interval 1.8 to 432.9).

Although this represents a very large and potentially alarming increased risk compared to the general population, the absolute risk of having a child with Beckwith–Wiedemann syndrome is very low. During the study period 14 894 children were born following IVF treatment in Victoria such that the absolute risk of having a liveborn baby with Beckwith–Wiedemann syndrome when IVF is used can be estimated as 4 in 14 894 or approximately 1 in every 4000 births. Whilst for an individual couple considering treatment the small absolute risk of having a child with

Beckwith–Wiedemann syndrome might not be of major consideration, given the very high risk, research into imprinting disorders and ART may prove very helpful in furthering our understanding of the etiology of adverse health outcomes in these children.

CONCLUSIONS

Properly conducted and appropriately sized cohort studies are the cornerstone of our understanding of health outcomes for children born following ART. The value of the results from such studies lies in the contribution they make to our understanding of the outcomes that children born following ART may experience and how the outcomes might have occurred. The results of these studies contribute important information for use in counseling and managing the expectations of couples considering treatment. In addition, the results aid our understanding of the biological basis of infertility; they aid our understanding of the effects that infertility and its related biological phenomena have on child health; and aid our understanding of the direct impact that the treatment processes involved may have upon the children born. Untangling treatment effects from the effects of infertility is the challenge for the future, and this will require well-designed cohort studies. We suggest that epidemiologists have an important contribution to make to the design, conduct and interpretation of these types of study to avoid some of the common mistakes illustrated in this chapter.

ACKNOWLEDGMENTS

Jennifer Kurinczuk is partially funded by a National Public Health Career Scientist Award from the Department of Health and NHS R&D (PHCS 022) and partially funded by the grant from the Department of Health to the National Perinatal Epidemiology Unit. Michèle Hansen is supported by a research grant (211930) from the National Health and Medical Research Council of Australia and Carol Bower is supported by a research fellowship (353628) from the same source.

REFERENCES

1. Cox GF, Bürger J, Lip V, et al. Intracytoplasmic sperm injection may increase the risk of imprinting defects. Am J Hum Genet 2002; 71: 162–4

2. Schieve LA, Rasmussen SA, Buck GM, et al. Are children born after assisted reproductive technology at increased risk for adverse health outcomes? Obstet Gynecol 2004; 103: 1154–63

3. Dhont M, De Sutter P, Ruyssinck G, et al. Perinatal outcome of pregnancies after assisted reproduction: a case–control study. Am J Obstet Gynecol 1999; 181: 688–95

4. Jackson RA, Gibson K, Wu YW, et al. Perinatal outcomes in singletons following in vitro fertilization: a meta-analysis. Obstet Gynecol 2004; 103: 551–63

5. Helmerhorst FM, Perquin DA, Donker D, et al. Perinatal outcome of singletons and twins after assisted conception: a systematic review of controlled studies. Br Med J 2004; 328: 261–5

6. Anthony S, Buitendijk SE, Dorrepaal CA, et al. Congenital malformations in 4224 children conceived after IVF. Hum Reprod 2002; 17: 2089–95

7. Bonduelle M, Legein J, Buysse A, et al. Prospective follow-up study of 423 children born after intracytoplasmic sperm injection. Hum Reprod 1996; 11: 1558–64

8. Kurinczuk JJ, Bower C. Birth defects in infants conceived by intracytoplasmic sperm injection: an alternative interpretation. Br Med J 1997; 315: 1260–5

9. Rimm AA, Katayama AC, Diaz M, et al. A meta-analysis of controlled studies comparing major malformation rates in IVF and ICSI infants with naturally conceived children. J Assist Reprod Genet 2004; 21: 437–43

10. Hansen M, Bower C, Milne E, et al. Assisted reproductive technologies and the risk of birth defects – a systematic review. Hum Reprod 2005; 20: 328–38

11. Verlaenen H, Cammu H, Derde MP, et al. Singleton pregnancy after in vitro fertilization: expectations and outcome. Obstet Gynecol 1995; 86: 906–10

12. Sutcliffe AG, D'Souza SW, Cadman J, et al. Outcome in children from cryopreserved embryos. Arch Dis Child 1995; 72: 290–3

13. Sutcliffe AG, D'Souza SW, Cadman J, et al. Minor congenital anomalies, major congenital anomalies and development in children conceived from cryopreserved embryos. Hum Reprod 1995; 10: 3332–7

14. Hansen M, Kurinczuk J, Bower C, et al. The risk of major birth defects after intracytoplasmic sperm injection and in vitro fertilization. N Engl J Med 2002; 346: 725–30

15. Rothman KJ, Greenland S. Types of epidemiologic studies. In: Rothman KJ, Greenland S, eds. Modern Epidemiology, 2nd edn. Philadelphia: Lippincott Williams and Wilkins, 1998: 67–78

16. Bowen JR, Gibson FL, Leslie GI, et al. Medical and developmental outcome at 1 year for children conceived by intracytoplasmic sperm injection. Lancet 1998; 351: 1529–34

17. Bonduelle M, Liebaers I, Deketelaere V, et al. Neonatal data on a cohort of 2889 infants born after ICSI (1991–1999) and of 2995 infants born after IVF (1983–1999). Hum Reprod 2002; 17: 671–94

18. Rothman KJ, Greenland S. Accuracy considerations in study design. In Rothman KJ, Greenland S, eds. Modern Epidemiology, 2nd edn. Philadelphia: Lippincott Williams and Wilkins, 1998: 115–34

19. Koivurova S, Hartikainen A-L, Sovio U, et al. Growth, psychomotor develop-
    ment and morbidity up to 3 years of age in children born after IVF. Hum
    Reprod 2003; 18: 2328–36
20. Gissler M, Malin Silverio M, Hemminki E. In-vitro fertilization pregnancies
    and perinatal health in Finland 1991–1993. Hum Reprod 1995; 10: 1856–61
21. Boyd P, Armstrong B, Dolk H, et al. Congenital anomaly surveillance in Eng-
    land – ascertainment deficiencies in the national system. Br Med J 2005; 330:
    27–9
22. Buck Louis GM, Schisterman EF, Dukic VM, et al. Research hurdles compli-
    cating the analysis of infertility treatment and child health. Hum Reprod 2005;
    20: 12–18
23. Breslow NE, Day NE. Statistical Methods in Cancer Research, vol 1. The
    analysis of Case–Control Studies. Lyon: International Agency for Research on
    Cancer, 1980: 84–119
24. Kupper LL, Palmer LJ. Matching. In: Elston R, Olsen J, Palmer L, eds. Biosta-
    tistical Genetics and Genetic Epidemiology. Chichester: John Wiley and Sons,
    2002: 518–23
25. Koudstaal J, Bruinse HW, Helmerhorst FM, et al. Obstetric outcome of twin
    pregnancies after in-vitro fertilization: a matched control study in four Dutch
    university hospitals. Hum Reprod 2000; 15: 935–40
26. Ombelet W, Peeraer K, De Sutter P, et al. Perinatal outcome of ICSI pregnan-
    cies compared with a matched group of natural conception pregnancies in
    Flanders (Belgium): a cohort study. Reprod Biomed Online 2005; 11: 244–53
27. Clarke M, Clayton D. The design and interpretation of case–control studies of
    perinatal mortality. Am J Epidemiol 1981; 113: 636–45
28. Pinborg A, Loft A, Nyboe Andersen A. Neonatal outcome in a Danish national
    cohort of 8602 children born after in vitro fertilization or intracytoplasmic
    sperm injection: the role of twin pregnancy. Acta Obstet Gynecol Scand 2004;
    83: 1070–8
29. Kurinczuk JJ, Hansen M, Bower C. The risk of birth defects in children born
    after assisted reproductive technologies. Curr Opin Obstet Gynaecol 2004; 16:
    201–9
30. Doyle P, Bunch KJ, Beral V, et al. Cancer incidence in children conceived with
    assisted reproduction technology. Lancet 1998; 352: 452–53
31. Rothman KJ, Greenland S. Approaches to statistical analysis. In Rothman KJ,
    Greenland S, eds. Modern Epidemiology, 2nd edn. Philadelphia: Lippincott
    Williams and Wilkins, 1998: 183–99
32. Morin NC, Wirth FH, Johnson DH, et al. Congenital malformations and psy-
    chosocial development in children conceived by in vitro fertilization. J Pediatr
    1989; 115: 222–7
33. Bruinsma F, Venn A, Lancaster P, et al. Incidence of cancer in children born
    after in-vitro fertilization. Hum Reprod 2000; 15: 604–7
34. Halliday J, Oke K, Breheny S, et al. Beckwith–Wiedemann syndrome and IVF:
    a case–control study. Am J Hum Genet 2004; 75: 526–8

Chapter 3

Congenital anomalies
after assisted reproduction

Christina Bergh and Ulla-Britt Wennerholm

INTRODUCTION

It is well established that children born after *in vitro* fertilization (IVF) have poorer outcomes than spontaneously conceived children, mainly depending on the high rate of multiple births and associated prematurity[1-6]. Other potential risks include an increased rate of malformations after assisted reproductive technology (ART). Lancaster's study from the 1980s was the first to report a higher prevalence of neural tube defects and transposition of the great vessels among IVF children[7]. Further studies were mostly reassuring as regards congenital malformations in children born after conventional IVF. However, comparisons were most often made with the expected outcome in the general population rather than with defined control groups. Controlled studies have been published more recently, where comparisons have been made with matched controls. In recent years large registry studies have also been published, comparing ART children with the general population before and after adjusting for parental confounders. Concerns have been raised that ART might increase the malformation rate in offspring, particularly after intracytoplasmic sperm injection (ICSI). The reason for these concerns is that the ICSI technique makes use of sperm bypassing natural selection, and thereby makes it possible for genetic material from otherwise incompetent spermatozoa to be transmitted. The technique itself is invasive and may interact with delicate procedures close to the meiotic spindle. It is also known that men with severe oligozoospermia have an increased rate of chromosomal aberrations[8,9]. Other potential risks, which also apply to IVF, include gonadotropin stimulation, the oocyte aspiration procedure and the culture condition.

The aim of this chapter is to summarize the present knowledge concerning malformations after assisted reproduction and particularly to discuss whether ART children have an increased risk of malformations in comparison with spontaneously conceived children and, if so, whether this increased risk could be related to the ART procedure or whether it is mainly related to parental characteristics, i.e. whether it disappears after adjusting for known confounders.

We searched PubMed and Cochrane databases for relevant articles published up to September 2005. The following keywords were used: *in vitro fertilization; IVF; intracytoplasmic sperm injection; ICSI; cryopreservation; malformation rate; birth defects.* When there were overlapping data, the most recent publication was chosen for studies listed in Table 3.1[10–17].

METHODOLOGICAL PROBLEMS

It is clear that many papers on malformations after ART have severe methodological limitations, e.g. selection for inclusion of children poorly described; inadequate description of when and by whom assessment was done; assessors not blinded to conception status; different methods used for malformation assessments for ART children and control group; different length of follow-up between groups; no/inadequate information about those who did not participate; ascertainment bias, etc.[18].

Another major problem is the definition of malformations. Major congenital malformations are anatomical defects or chromosomal abnormalities that are present at birth and are either fatal or significantly affect the individual's function or appearance. They occur in the general population in 2–3% of all births, with about 0.5–0.6% consisting of chromosomal abnormalities[19,20]. Despite development of an international classification system, the International Classification of Diseases (ICD-9 and ICD-10), different countries and reports do not classify malformations in exactly the same way.

POPULATION-BASED REGISTRY STUDIES

Population-based registry studies of malformations have the clear advantage of large sample sizes, enabling cross-linkage research, not requiring patient contact and minimizing losses to follow-up. By far the largest published registry study is the recently published report from Sweden[17]. This study covers the period 1992–2001. Among 16 280 identified IVF children, 811 had a diagnosis of a congenital malformation in the Swedish

Medical Birth Registry (SMBR) (5.0%), while among all children registered in the SMBR during this period (a total of 2 039 943 children), 80 881 had such a diagnosis (4.0%). The crude risk ratio was thus 1.26 (Table 3.1). Among the malformed IVF children 535 (3.3%) had a severe malformation, while the figure for the general population was 45 892 (2.2%), crude risk ratio 1.46. Although other population registries (the Swedish Registry of Congenital Malformations and the Swedish Hospital Discharge Registry) were checked for malformations as well, only the SMBR was used for comparison, owing to incompleteness for non-IVF children in those other registries. The crude odds ratios were thus both significantly increased. The increase disappeared, however, after adjustment for confounders: maternal age, parity, known years of infertility, plurality and smoking. Since this was such a large population, subdivision according to the technique used was done, i.e. standard IVF, ICSI, frozen embryos, epididymal and testicular sperm. The malformation rates varied between 2.7% and 9.1% when all malformations were included (i.e. also malformations detected in other population registries). No significant difference was noted for any technique in comparison with standard IVF. For some specific malformations, i.e. anencephaly, spina bifida, cardiovascular defects, orofacial clefts and alimentary tract atresia, a significant increase in observed versus expected numbers was noted. The only malformation that was increased in ICSI versus IVF was hypospadias. Only two conditions showed significantly higher rates of multiple births, anencephaly and hydrocephaly. Two infants with malformations that have been associated with imprinting anomalies were identified, one child with Prader–Willi syndrome and one child with Russel–Silver syndrome.

The overall conclusion from this large study was that children born after IVF have a modest but significantly increased rate of congenital malformations, similar after IVF and ICSI. This seemed to a large extent to be due to parental characteristics, and for hydrocephaly to multiple births. The extra risk for the individual couple was, however, very low.

In an Australian registry study[16], the prevalences of major birth defects in children born after ICSI ($n = 301$), conventional IVF ($n = 837$) and spontaneous conception ($n = 4000$) and detected by 1 year of age were 8.6%, 9.0% and 4.2%, respectively. After adjustment for confounders such as maternal age, parity and sex, the children born after ART were still twice as likely to have a birth defect as children born after natural conception. More defects in infants conceived through assisted reproduction were also observed when only singleton or term singleton births were considered. Increases in risk were found for most categories of defect, and the differences were significant for musculoskeletal and cardiovascular defects. Although the rate of birth defects after ART in this study was alarmingly

Table 3.1 Population-based registry studies on malformations after assisted reproductive technology (ART)

Authors, year	Country	Study population (n)	ART	Malformations (%)	All/ major/ minor	Crude/ adjusted/ matched	OR/RR	95% CI
Beral and Doyle, 1990[10]	UK	1581	IVF, GIFT	2.2	Major	Adjusted	1.11	0.79–1.43
Addor et al., 1998[11]	Switzerland	148	IVF, other	4.7	All	Crude	2.01	0.93–4.38
Westergaard et al., 1999[12]	Denmark	2245	IVF, ICSI	4.8	All	Matched	1.04	0.78–1.39
Dhont et al., 1999[13]	Belgium	3048, singletons	IVF, GIFT	2.8	All	Matched	1.36	0.97–1.93
Anthony et al., 2002[14]	The Netherlands	4224	IVF, ICSI	3.2	All	Crude/ adjusted	1.20/1.03	1.01–1.43/ 0.86–1.23
Ludwig and Katalanic, 2002[15]	Germany	3372	ICSI	8.6	Major	Crude	1.25	1.11–1.40
Hansen et al., 2002[16]	Australia	1138	IVF, ICSI	8.9	Major	Adjusted	2.04	1.50–2.77
Källen et al., 2005[17]	Sweden	16 280	IVF, ICSI	5.0	All	Crude/ adjusted	1.26/0.86	1.18–1.36/ 0.70–1.05

IVF, in vitro fertilization; GIFT, gamete intra-Fallopian transfer; ICSI, intracytoplasmic sperm injection high, the study population was quite small and there were also some demographic differences, such as ethnic origin and place of residence, which could have influenced the results.

A Dutch study[14] of 4224 children born after IVF showed a crude odds ratio (OR) of 1.20 (95% CI 1.01–1.43) for the risk of any malformation in IVF children. After adjustment for maternal age, parity and ethnicity, the OR was lower and no longer significant (Table 3.1). A German prospective, multicenter, controlled study reported 8.6% major malformations (in liveborns, stillborns, spontaneous and induced abortions from the 16th week of pregnancy) in the ICSI cohort and 6.9% in the spontaneous control group. However, no information was given about individuals who refused to participate in this study[15].

In a Danish registry study 2245 IVF children were compared with a matched control group from the Danish Medical Birth Registry and with all births in the Danish Medical Birth Registry[12]. In all, 107 (4.8%) of IVF children and 103 (4.6%) in the control group were born with malformations as compared to 2.8% in the background population. The results indicated that it is more the characteristics of the patients and multiple pregnancy, than the assisted reproductive technology that determines the fetal risks of IVF pregnancies as compared to the background population. In a recent registry study from Israel[21], congenital malformations in ART children during two time periods were compared to children born after spontaneous conception. The study populations were 278 and 1632 ART children and the control populations included 31 007 and 53 208 children. Major malformations were found in 9.35% in the first and 9.0% in the second IVF cohort which were 2.3-fold and 1.75-fold higher than the figures for the control population.

CASE–CONTROL STUDIES

In two Dutch studies[22,23], 307 singletons and 96 twins after IVF were compared with 307 and 96 control pregnancies after elaborate matching for an extensive number of maternal characteristics, as well as for birth hospital (Table 3.2)[21-38]. In the singleton cohorts, in both groups seven children (2.3%) had congenital malformations and in the twin cohorts seven (3.7%), while five (2.6%) malformations were reported for IVF and controls. In an Australian cohort study 89 ICSI children, 84 IVF children and 80 children born after spontaneous conception were investigated at 1 year of age[31]. There were no significant differences in the incidence of major malformations amongst the ICSI (4.5%), IVF (3.6%) and naturally conceived children (5%). In a case–control study from the UK, 208 singleton

Table 3.2 Case–control studies on malformation rate after assisted reproductive technology (ART)

Authors, year	Country	Study population (n)	ART	Malformation rate (%)	All/ major/ minor	Crude, adjusted/ matched	OR	95% CI
Morin et al., 1989[24]	USA	83	IVF	2.4	Major	Matched	2.27	0.12–135.45
Sutcliffe et al., 1995[25]	UK	91	IVF	3.3	Major	Matched	1.40	0.20–8.50
Tanbo et al., 1995[26]	Norway	355	IVF, GIFT	2.0	All	Matched	1.16	0.38–3.30
Verlaenen et al., 1995[27]	Belgium	140	IVF, singletons	5.7	Minor	Matched	7.15	0.59–infinity
Nassar et al., 1996[28]	Egypt	128	IVF	NA	Major	Crude	1.60	0.21–12.12
D'Souza et al., 1997[29]	UK	278	IVF	2.5	Major	Matched	15.39	1.90–infinity
Fisch et al., 1997[30]	Israel	100	IVF	NA	Major	Crude	4.60	1.86–9.95
Bowen et al., 1998[31]	Australia	173	IVF, ICSI	4.0	Major	Crude	0.80	0.20–3.85
Koudstaal et al., 2000[22]	The Netherlands	307	IVF-singleton	2.3	All	Matched	1.00	0.29–3.39
Koudstaal et al., 2000[23]	The Netherlands	192	IVF-twins	3.7	All	Matched	1.42	0.38–5.76
Sutcliffe et al., 2001[32]	UK	208	ICSI, singletons	4.8	Major	Matched	1.06	0.39–2.92

continued

Table 3.2 *Continued*

Authors, year	Country	Study population (n)	ART	Malformation rate (%)	All/ major/ minor	Crude, adjusted/ matched	OR	95% CI
Zuppa et al., 2001[33]	Italy	32	IVF, GIFT (twins)	NA	Major	Crude	2.42	0.04–31.08
Wang et al., 2002[34]	Australia	1019	IVF, ICSI, GIFT	4.3	All	Matched	0.95	0.61–1.49
Isaksson et al., 2002[35]	Finland	109	IVF, ICSI	5.5	Major	Matched	1.61	0.51–4.33
Koivurova et al., 2002[36]	Finland	304	IVF	6.6	All	Matched	1.61	0.51–4.33
Sutcliffe et al., 2003[37]	Australia	56	ICSI	8.9	Major	Matched	0.67	0.14–3.15
Zadori et al., 2003[38]	Hungary	262	IVF	1.9	Major	Matched	1.68	0.32–10.92
Merlob et al., 2005[21]	Israel	278	IVF, ICSI	9.1	Major	Crude	2.1	1.66–2.28

IVF, *in vitro* fertilization; GIFT, gamete intra-Fallopian transfer; ICSI, intracytoplasmic sperm injection children conceived by ICSI and a control group of 221 normally conceived children were studied[32]. The control children were matched to cases as closely as possible according to social class, maternal education, region, sex and race. The rate of congenital malformations was similar in the two groups: 4.8% and 4.5%, respectively.

In a Swedish study[39], the incidence of malformations was investigated in 1139 ICSI children and compared with all births in the Medical Birth Registry. Of the ICSI children 7.6% had an anomaly, of which 4.1% were major. The OR for ICSI children for having any major or minor malformation was 1.75 (95% CI 1.19–2.58). After adjusting for confounders, however, the OR was reduced to 1.19 and was no longer significant. The only specific malformation found in excess in children born after ICSI was hypospadias (RR 3.0, 95% CI 1.09–6.50) which might be related to paternal subfertility. This excess in hypospadias in ICSI infants was also confirmed in the larger Swedish registry study[17]. In an American study of 278 IVF children, 2.5% had a major malformation, as compared to none in the controls[29].

In a Finnish study, 340 IVF children were compared with 569 controls from the general population, randomly selected from the Finnish Medical Birth Registry and matched for sex, year of birth, area of residence, parity, maternal age and social class[36]. Plurality-matched controls were also included. A four-fold increase in heart malformations was found among IVF children as compared to controls from the general population (OR 4.0, 95% CI 1.4–11.7). However, after stratifying for plurality, the OR was no longer significant. No significant increase was noted for other malformations. In another Finnish case–control study[35], the outcome among women with unexplained infertility and IVF (92 children) was compared to matched spontaneous controls (545 children). The matching variables were maternal age, parity, year of birth, mother's residence and plurality. A second control group included all IVF children born during the study period (n = 2853). The rate of major congenital malformation was 7.2% in IVF singletons and 3.5% in controls (NS). No significant differences were found between twins.

MALFORMATION RATE IN ICSI VERSUS IVF

In the large Swedish registry study[17], 4949 ICSI children and 11 283 IVF children were included. The malformation rate was similar in the two groups: 8.6% and 8.1%, respectively. In the ICSI/epididymal sperm group, ten out of 135 children had a malformation (7.4%) and in the ICSI/ testicular sperm group 11 out of 147 children (7.5%) did. Thus, although few such children were included, there was no indication of an increased malformation rate after using surgically retrieved sperm. Ludwig and co-workers[15] found no increase in malformations in the groups using epididymal (1/26; 3.8%) or testicular sperm (21/229; 9.2%) compared to ejaculated sperm (8.4%). The Belgian group has, since the beginning of IVF/ICSI, performed a meticulous follow-up of children born after ART, including data on neonatal outcome and congenital malformations during pregnancy and at birth. The latest report includes 2889 children born after ICSI and 2995 children born after IVF[40]. The total malformation rate, taking into account major malformations in stillborns, terminations and live-borns was 4.2% in the ICSI group and 4.6% in the IVF group. The malformation rate in the ICSI cohort was not related to sperm origin or sperm quality[40]. However, their study had no control group of spontaneously conceived children (Table 3.3)[16,17,40,41].

META-ANALYSIS OF MALFORMATIONS IN ART CHILDREN

Four meta-analyses have been published recently (Table 3.4)[6,42–44]. The Hansen meta-analysis[43] specifically addressed malformations after IVF/ICSI in studies published up to March 2003. A total of 51 papers were identified and eventually 25 studies were assessed, where no overlap in patient material was found. Only seven papers were considered to be appropriate for inclusion in the meta-analysis. The majority of these were population based with a clear definition of a birth defect. Most had large sample sizes and birth defects were ascertained without knowledge of conception status. The pooled OR for a major malformation, including these seven studies, was 1.40 (95% CI 1.28–1.53) while the pooled OR when all 25 studies were included was 1.29 (95% CI 1.21–1.37).

A Norwegian meta-analysis[44] compared malformations in ICSI versus IVF in studies published up until May 2002. Out of more than 400 articles only 22 studies contained relevant data on ICSI children. Exclusions were performed for overlapping data, for non-prospective design and for studies not taking abortions into account. Four prospective studies remained and were included in the meta-analysis (Table 3.3). Reported prevalences of major malformations varied from 3.0% to 9.0% across studies. Of the four studies included in the Norwegian meta-analysis only one estimated an increased risk of major malformations after ICSI as compared to standard IVF[45]: 7.1% versus 5.3%. However, in a later publication by the same authors and including a larger number of children, this difference in malformations between ICSI and IVF was no longer noted[17]. The pooled

Table 3.3 Malformations after assisted reproductive technology (ART): intracytoplasmic sperm injection (ICSI) versus *in vitro* fertilization (IVF)

Authors, year	Country	Pregnancy inclusion criteria, weeks	Induced abortions included	Number of ICSI children	Children with malformations, ICSI	Number of IVF children	Children with malformations, IVF	RR/OR (95% CI)
Bonduelle et al., 2002[40]	Belgium	16	Yes	2889	121 (4.2%)	2995	135 (4.5%)	0.93 (0.73–1.18)
Hansen et al., 2002[16]	Australia	21	Yes	301	26 (8.6%)	837	75 (9.0%)	0.96 (0.63–1.48)
Oldereid et al., 2003[41]	Norway	16	Yes	553	17 (3.1%)	1731	52 (3.0%)	1.02 (0.97–1.28)
Källen et al., 2005[17]	Sweden	28	No	4949	428 (8.6%)	11283	913 (8.1%)	1.00 (0.74–1.36)

Table 3.4 Meta-analysis of malformations after assisted reproductive technology (ART)

Authors, year	No. of studies included	No. of ART children included	Comparison	Plurality	OR/RR	95% CI
Rimm et al., 2004[42]	19	35 758	IVF/ICSI vs. spontaneously conceived children	All	1.29	1.01–1.67
Hansen et al., 2005[43]	7/25	16 038/28 638	IVF/ICSI vs. spontaneously conceived children	All	1.40/1.29	1.28–1.53/ 1.21–1.37
McDonald et al., 2005[6]	7	4031	IVF/ICSI vs. spontaneously conceived children	Singleton	1.41	1.06–1.88
Lie et al., 2005[44]	4	5395/12 786	ICSI/IVF	All	1.12	0.97–1.28

IVF, in vitro fertilization; ICSI, intracytoplasmic sperm injection risk ratio (RR) for a major malformation in the Norwegian meta-analysis was 1.12 (95% CI 0.97–1.28).

In a meta-analysis from the USA[42], in which 19 studies satisfied the selection criteria, the rate of major malformations ranged from 0 to 9.5% for IVF, 1.1 to 9.7% for ICSI and 0 to 6.9% for controls. When data from 16 studies involving 28 524 IVF children and 2 520 988 spontaneously conceived children, and seven studies involving 7234 ICSI children and 978 078 controls were pooled, an overall OR for the 19 studies of 1.29 (95% CI 1.01–1.67) was found.

In the most recent meta-analysis from Canada[6], singletons from IVF/ICSI were found to have a significantly increased OR for congenital malformations (OR 1.41; 95% CI 1.06–1.88).

CHROMOSOMAL ABERRATIONS

In national cohort studies from Scandinavia[12,45], including mainly IVF children, no increases in chromosomal aberrations were reported. However, some early reports from The Netherlands indicated an alarmingly high rate of chromosomal aberrations in studies with small numbers of patients included[46,47]. The largest study from Belgium showed that, among 1 586 prenatal tests, 3.0% were abnormal[48]. Of these, 1.4% of chromosomal aberrations were inherited from one of the parents. In another study, from Egypt[49], abnormal karyotypes were found in 3.5% of 430 ICSI babies, as compared to none in 430 naturally conceived babies. Based on these results, there seems to be a moderate excess of chromosomal aberrations following ICSI, as compared to approximately 1% described in neonatal populations[19,20]. However, some of the excess risk seems to be related to parental characteristics and not to the ICSI technique used (Table 3.5)[15,39,46–50].

CONCLUSIONS AND COMMENTS

Data from controlled studies seem to indicate a slight increase in major malformations in children born after IVF/ICSI as compared with naturally conceived children. There seems to be no difference in risk between more invasive techniques (ICSI) or less invasive ones (conventional IVF). Whether the increased risk is attributable to the *in vitro* culture technique or the ovarian stimulation procedure, or whether infertility *per se* is a risk factor, still remains to be elucidated. Studies published to date suggest the

Table 3.5 Chromosomal aberrations among fetuses/babies conceived from intracytoplasmic sperm injection (ICSI) reported in the literature

Authors, year	Country	No. of tested ICSI-conceived fetuses/babies	Abnormal de novo (n, %)	Inherited aberrations (n, %)	All aberrations (n, %)
In't Veld et al., 1995[46]	The Netherlands	15	5 (33.3)	0	5 (33.3)
Van Opstal et al., 1997[47]	The Netherlands	71	9 (12.7)	0	9 (12.7)
Loft et al., 1999[50]	Denmark	206	6 (2.9)	1 (0.5)	7 (3.4)
Wennerholm et al., 2000[39]	Sweden	149	2 (1.3)	2 (1.3)	4 (2.6)
Aboulghar et al., 2001[49]	Egypt	430	NA	NA	15 (3.5)
Bonduelle et al., 2002[48]	Belgium	1586	25 (1.6)	22 (1.4)	47 (3.0)
Ludwig et al., 2002[15]	Germany	830	NA	NA	28 (3.3)

latter explanation; when risk has been adjusted for parental characteristics the risk decreases and is no longer significant.

That subfertility *per se* might be a risk factor for poor obstetric outcome is supported by several studies. A recent study from the UK[51] concluded that subfertile women were at higher risk of obstetric complications, which persist after adjusting for age and parity. There were no differences between treatment-related and treatment-independent pregnancies. Similar data have been published from Denmark[52,53], where time to pregnancy of more than 1 year was associated with an increased risk of poor outcome, including preterm birth.

Regarding the risk of major malformations in spontaneously conceived pregnancies in subfertile women, a Swedish study from 1991 analyzed a cohort of 384 589 children from Sweden 1983–1986. In all, 7.8% showed subfertility, defined by time to conceive of more than 12 months. No IVF/ICSI treatment was included, but 24% had used clomiphene citrate. In addition to increased risks of preterm birth, the risk of major malformations was also higher, depending on time to pregnancy, after 5 years or more as compared to less time; the OR was 1.18 (95% CI 1.01–1.37)[54].

The absolute risk and risk difference for a major congenital malformation are, however, low and probably acceptable for the couples concerned. Most children born after ART are healthy, particularly if we turn to single embryo transfer for a majority of the patients, thereby decreasing the multiple birth rates dramatically, as recently shown for the Scandinavian countries[55,56].

REFERENCES

1. Bergh T, Ericsson A, Hillensjö T, et al. Deliveries and children born after in-vitro fertilisation in Sweden 1982–1995: a retrospective cohort study. Lancet 1999; 354: 1579–85

2. Schieve LA, Meikle SF, Ferre C, et al. Low and very low birth weight in infants conceived with the use of assisted reproduction technology. N Engl J Med 2002; 346: 731–7

3. Helmerhorst FM, Perquin DA, Donker D, et al. Perinatal outcomes in singletons and twins after assisted conception: a systematic review of controlled studies. Br Med J 2004; 328: 261–5

4. Jackson RA, Gibson KA, Wu YW, et al. Perinatal outcomes in singletons following in vitro fertilization: a meta-analysis. Obstet Gynecol 2004; 103: 551–63

5. Wennerholm UB, Bergh C. Outcome of IVF pregnancies. Fetal Matern Med Rev 2004; 15: 27–57

6. McDonald SD, Murphy K, Beyene J, et al. Perinatal outcomes of singleton pregnancies achieved by in vitro fertilization: a systematic review and meta-analysis. J Obstet Gynaecol Can 2005; 27: 449–59

7. Lancaster PA. Obstetric outcome. Clin Obstet Gynaecol 1985; 12: 847–64

8. de Braekeleer M, Dao TN. Cytogenetic studies in male infertility: a review. Hum Reprod 1991; 6: 245–50

9. Aittomäki K, Bergh C, Hazekamp J, et al. Genetics and assisted reproduction technology. Acta Obstet Gynecol Scand 2005; 84: 463–73

10. Beral V, Doyle P. Births in Great Britain resulting from assisted conception, 1978–87 (MRC Working Party on Children conceived by In Vitro Fertilisation). Br Med J 1990; 300: 1229–33

11. Addor V, Santos-Eggimann B, Fawer CL, et al. Impact of infertility treatments on health of newborns. Fertil Steril 1998; 69: 210–15

12. Westergaard HB, Johansen AM, Erb K, et al. Danish National in-vitro fertilization Registry 1994 and 1995: a controlled study of births, malformations and cytogenetic findings. Hum Reprod 1999; 14: 1896–902

13. Dhont M, De Sutter P, Ruyssinck G, et al. Perinatal outcome of pregnancies after assisted reproduction: a case–control study. Am J Obstet Gynecol 1999; 181: 688–95

14. Anthony S, Buitendijk SE, Dorrepaal CA, et al. Congenital malformations in 4224 children conceived after IVF. Hum Reprod 2002; 17: 2089–95

15. Ludwig M, Katalanic A. Malformation rate in fetuses and children conceived after ICSI: results of a prospective cohort study. RBM online 2002: 5: 171–8

16. Hansen M, Kurinczuk JJ, Bower C, et al. The risk of major birth defects after intracytoplasmic sperm injection and in vitro fertilization. N Engl J Med 2002; 346: 725–30

17. Källen B, Finnström O, Nygren KG, et al. In vitro fertilization (IVF) in Sweden: Risk for congenital malformations after different IVF methods. Birth Defects Res (Part A) Clin Mol Teratol 2005; 73: 162–9

18. Simpson JL. Registration of congenital anomalies in ART population: pitfalls. Hum Reprod 1996; (Suppl 4): 81–8

19. Nielsen J, Wohlert M. Chromosome abnormalities found among 34,910 newborn children: results from a 13-year incidence study in Arhus, Denmark. Hum Genet 1991; 87: 81–3

20. Jacobs PA, Browne C, Gregson N, et al. Estimates of the frequency of chromosome abnormalities detectable in unselected newborns using moderate levels of banding. J Med Genet 1992; 29: 103–8

21. Merlob P, Sapir O, Sulkes J, et al. The prevalence of major congenital malformations during two periods of time, 1986–1994 and 1994–2002 in newborns conceived by assisted reproduction technology. Eur J Med Genet 2005; 48: 5–11

22. Koudstaal J, Braat DD, Bruinse HW, et al. Obstetric outcome of singleton pregnancies after IVF: a matched control study in four Dutch university hospitals. Hum Reprod 2000; 15: 1819–25

23. Koudstaal J, Bruinse HW, Helmerhorst FM, et al. Obstetric outcome of twin pregnancies after in-vitro fertilization: a matched control study in four Dutch university hospitals. Hum Reprod 2000; 15: 935–40

24. Morin NC, Wirth FH, Johnson DH, et al. Congenital malformations and psychosocial development in children conceived by in vitro fertilization. J Pediatr 1989; 115: 222–7

25. Sutcliffe AG, D'Souza SW, Cadman J, et al. Minor congenital anomalies, major congenital malformations and development in children conceived from cryopreserved embryos. Hum Reprod 1995; 10: 3332–7

26. Tanbo T, Dale PO, Lunde O, et al. Obstetric outcome in singleton pregnancies after assisted reproduction. Obstet Gynecol 1995; 86: 188–92

27. Verlaenen H, Cammu H, Derde MP, et al. Singleton pregnancy after in vitro fertilization: expectations and outcome. Obstet Gynecol 1995; 86: 906–10

28. Nassar S, Boutros J, Aboulghar H, et al. Perinatal outcome after in vitro fertilization and spontaneous pregnancy: a comparative study. Middle East Fertil Soc J 1996; 1: 151–8

29. D'Souza SW, Rivlin E, Cadman J, et al. Children conceived by in vitro fertilisation after fresh embryo transfer. Arch Dis Child 1997: 76: F70–4

30. Fisch B, Harel L, Kaplan B, et al. Neonatal assessment of babies conceived by in vitro fertilization. J Perinatol 1997; 17: 473–6

31. Bowen JR, Gibson FL, Leslie GI, et al. Medical and development outcome at 1 year for children conceived by intracytoplasmic sperm injection. Lancet 1998; 351: 1529–34

32. Sutcliffe AG, Taylor B, Saunders K, et al. Outcome in the second year of life after in vitro fertilisation by intracytoplasmic sperm injection: a UK case–control study. Lancet 2001; 357: 2080–4

33. Zuppa AA, Maragliano G, Scapillati ME, et al. Neonatal outcome of spontaneous and assisted twin pregnancies. Eur J Obstet Gynecol Reprod Biol 2001; 95: 68–72

34. Wang JX, Norman RJ, Kristiansson P. The effect of various infertility treatments on the risk of preterm birth. Hum Reprod 2002; 17: 945–9

35. Isaksson R, Gissler M, Tiitinen A. Obstetric outcome among women with unexplained infertility after IVF: a matched case–control study. Hum Reprod 2002; 17: 1755–61

36. Koivurova S, Hartikainen AL, Gissler M, et al. Neonatal outcome and congenital malformations in children born after in-vitro fertilization. Hum Reprod 2002; 17: 1391–8

37. Sutcliffe AG, Saunders K, Mclachlan R, et al. A retrospective case–control study of development and other outcomes in a cohort of Australian children conceived by intracytoplasmic sperm injection compared with a similar group in the United Kingdom. Fertil Steril 2003; 79: 512–16

38. Zadori ZJ, Kozinszky Z, Orvos H, et al. The incidence of major birth defects following in vitro fertilization. J Assist Reprod Genet 2003; 20: 131–2

39. Wennerholm UB, Bergh C, Hamberger L, et al. Incidence of congenital malformations in children born after ICSI. Hum Reprod 2000; 15: 944–8

40. Bonduelle M, Liebaers I, Deketelaere V, et al. Neonatal data on a cohort of 2889 infants born after ICSI (1991–1999) and of 2995 infants born after IVF (1983–1999). Hum Reprod 2002; 17: 671–94

41. Oldereid NB, Äbyholm T, Tanbo T, et al. Congenital malformations in children born after assisted fertilization in Norway. Tidsk Nor Laegeforen 2003; 123: 269–9

42. Rimm AA, Katayama AC, Diaz M, et al. A meta-analysis of controlled studies comparing major malformation rates in IVF and ICSI infants with naturally conceived children. J Assist Reprod Genet 2004; 21: 437–43

43. Hansen M, Bower C, Milne E, et al. Assisted reproductive technologies and the risk of birth defects – a systematic review. Hum Reprod 2005; 20: 328–38

44. Lie RT, Lyngstadaas A, Örstavik KH, et al. Birth defects in children conceived by other IVF methods: a meta-analysis. Int J Epidemiol 2005; 34: 696–701

45. Ericson A, Källen B. Congenital malformations in infants born after IVF: a population-based study. Hum Reprod 2001; 16: 504–9

46. In't Veld P, Brandenburg H, Verhoeff A, et al. Sex chromosomal abnormalities and intracytoplasmic sperm injection. Lancet 1995; 346: 773

47. Van Opstal D, Los FJ, Ramlakhan S, et al. Determination of the parent of origin in nine cases of prenatal detected chromosome aberrations found after intracytoplasmic sperm injection. Hum Reprod 1997; 12: 682–6

48. Bonduelle M, Van Assche E, Joris H, et al. Prenatal testing in ICSI pregnancies: incidence of chromosomal anomalies in 1586 karyotypes and relation to sperm parameters. Hum Reprod 2002; 17: 2600–14

49. Aboulghar H, Aboulghar M, Mansour R, et al. A prospective controlled study of karyotyping for 430 consecutive babies conceived through intracytoplasmic sperm injection. Fertil Steril 2001; 76: 249–53

50. Loft A, Petersen K, Erb K, et al. A Danish national cohort of 730 infants born after intracytoplasmic sperm injection (ICSI) 1994–1997. Hum Reprod 1999; 14: 2143–8

51. Thomson F, Shanbhag S, Templeton A, et al. Obstetric outcome in women with subfertility. Br J Obstet Gynaecol 2005; 112: 632–7

52. Henriksen TB, Baird DD, Olsen J, et al. Time to pregnancy and preterm delivery. Obstet Gynecol 1997; 89: 594–9

53. Basso O, Baird DD. Infertility and preterm delivery, birth weight, and Caesarean section: a study within the Danish National Birth cohort. Hum Reprod 2003: 18: 2478–84

54. Ghazi HA, Spielberger C, Källen B. Delivery outcome after infertility – a registry study. Fertil Steril 1991; 55: 726–32

55. Bergh C. Single embryo transfer: a mini-review. Hum Reprod 2005; 20: 323–7

56. Bergh C, Thurin-Kjellberg A, Karlsröm PO. Ett ägg vid provrörsbefruktning. Läkartidningen 2005; 102: 3444–9

Chapter 4

Perinatal outcome
after assisted reproduction

Ulla-Britt Wennerholm and Christina Bergh

INTRODUCTION

More than 25 years have passed since the first 'test tube baby' was born[1]. Since then, more than one million children worldwide have been born after *in vitro* fertilization (IVF)[2]. In many industrialized countries, IVF children constitute 2–4% of all newborn babies[3].

The course and outcome of IVF pregnancies have been the subject of a considerable number of publications. Initially these were mainly descriptive studies concerning pregnancy outcome, but today more and more information is available from controlled studies and meta-analyses and about the long-term consequences for the children.

After conventional IVF was established, the cryopreservation technique was developed; the first baby produced after implementing this technique was born in 1984[4]. Next came intracytoplasmic sperm injection (ICSI), with the first baby born in 1992[5]. New and more advanced techniques are constantly being developed, making continuous surveillance of outcomes following assisted conception mandatory.

This chapter addresses the perinatal outcome after assisted conception focusing on the most recent data available. We have focused on preterm birth and low birth weight (LBW), which are the most important determinants of perinatal mortality and neonatal, infant and childhood morbidity.

We searched the PubMed and Cochrane databases for articles published before August 2005, using the following key words and subject terms: 'fertilization in vitro', 'in vitro fertilization', 'assisted reproduction', 'ICSI', 'intracytoplasmic sperm injection', 'microinjection' and 'obstetric outcome', 'perinatal outcome', 'perinatal care', 'neonatal outcome'.

MULTIPLE BIRTHS

Multiple births are now recognized as a major problem associated with assisted conception. Data from the large European and American registries of assisted reproduction show high multiple pregnancy rates after IVF and ICSI. The multiple birth rates have been fairly constant over the past decade and were, according to the latest reports, 25.5% and 35.4% for Europe[3] and the USA[6], respectively, much higher rates than in the general population, where multiple births constitute 1–2% of all births. Analyses of individual infants (rather than infant-sets or deliveries) indicate that 54% of infants born after assisted reproductive technology (ART) in the USA in 2001 were multiples, as compared with only 3% in the general population[6,7].

Multiple births are associated with considerable medical risk for the mother and offspring as well as incurring excess obstetric and neonatal costs. Multiple pregnancies are more likely to result in preterm birth, a LBW infant, infant death, congenital malformations and disability among survivors. The risks increase with the number of fetuses. Women carrying a multiple pregnancy have an increased risk of anemia, pregnancy-induced hypertension and pre-eclampsia, as well as maternal mortality. The birth is frequently more complicated with more surgical interventions and postpartum hemorrhaging. Therefore, when the general obstetric outcome in assisted conception is analyzed with singleton and multiple pregnancies combined, a more adverse outcome compared with the general population is to be expected. Table 4.1[8–12] shows clearly that preterm deliveries and LBW as well as perinatal mortality occur in much higher frequencies in assisted conception pregnancies than in the general population, the risk being around four- to five-fold for preterm birth and LBW.

The most important factor influencing the rate of multiple births in IVF is the number of embryos transferred. One way of preventing adverse outcome is therefore to limit the number of embryos transferred. In the early days of IVF, several embryos were transferred, often four or five. Some countries have now developed guidelines to limit the number of embryos transferred. In Germany, the maximum number of embryos for transfer in any treatment cycle is three, while in the UK the number of embryos has recently been limited to two[13]. In the Nordic countries dual embryo transfer (DET) has been the standard for several years. In Sweden, the change in clinical policy to reduce the number of embryos transferred from three to two led to a virtual disappearance of triplets and a reduction in twin deliveries from 29% in 1991 to 18.5% in 2001[14]. The risk of preterm birth after IVF was reduced by 70%. To further reduce twin deliveries, elective single embryo transfer (eSET) has been introduced in some

Table 4.1 General obstetric outcomes in assisted conception populations versus general populations

Author, country, year of publication	IVF (n)	Multiple pregnancy in IVF (%)	General population (n)	IVF <37 weeks (%)	General population <37 weeks (%)	IVF <2500 g (%)	General population <2500 g (%)	IVF perinatal mortality§ (‰)	General population perinatal mortality§ (‰)
MRC, UK, 1990[8]	1581	23.0	NA[a]	24.0[b]	6.0	32.0[b]	7.0	27.2[b]	9.8
Friedler, Israel, 1992[9]	1453	23.6	22778[c]	28.6	NA	23.8[c]	6.4	22.8[c]	13.0
Gissler, Finland, 1995[10]	1335	26.5	193048	24.7[d]	5.0	30.6[d]	3.9	29.3[d]	7.3
Rufat, France, 1994[11]	1669	27.0	NA	22.7[b]	5.6[e]	34.7[b]	5.2[e]	30.6[b]	NA
Bergh, Sweden, 1999[12]	5856	26.9	1505724	23.6[b]	5.1	21.3[b]	3.8	18[b]	6.6

§Definitions of perinatal mortality. MRC, stillbirth at 28 weeks or more and death in first 7 days; Friedler, stillbirth at 26 weeks or more and death in first 7 days; Bergh, stillbirth at 28 weeks or more and death in first 7 days. [a]Compared with all deliveries in England and Wales, without matching; [b]no statistics available; [c]p<0.05 compared with national census, without matching; [d]p<0.001 in comparison with all naturally conceived pregnancies in Finland during the same time period; [e]national statistics countries. The largest randomized controlled trial on eSET versus DET was initiated in Sweden[15]. In the SET group women received a single embryo transfer and, if there was no live birth, subsequently a frozen SET, whereas women in the DET group received a double embryo transfer on one occasion. This Scandinavian multicenter study showed that the SET group achieved a rate of live birth not substantially lower than was achieved with DET. The rates of multiple births in the two groups were 0.8% in SET and 34.5% in DET and consequently the rate of maternal and pediatric complications, especially preterm births, was lower in the SET group[16].

In a Belgian review, including four prospective randomized trials, one of which was an abstract from the Scandinavian multicenter study, the mean fresh pregnancy rate after SET in the four studies was 30.7%, with 2.2% twins, and after DET it was 47.6%, with 33.8% twins[17]. In a recent Cochrane review the effectiveness of two versus one embryo was evaluated. The results showed a clinical pregnancy rate in two versus one embryo transfer of odds ratio (OR) 2.16 (95% confidence interval (CI) 1.65–2.82), live birth rate OR 1.94 (95% CI 1.47–2.55) and multiple birth rate OR 23.55 (95% CI 8.00–69.29)[18]. The results were based on the same four randomized trials as in the Belgian review and were dominated by the Scandinavian study.

An overview of the implementation of SET in Sweden is presented in a recent publication[2]. Data for 2004 in Sweden showed an increased SET rate, a further reduction in multiple birth rate to 5% and an unchanged delivery rate[19].

It is evident that SET reduces the twin birth rate considerably and maintains an ongoing pregnancy rate of 30–40% per transfer. Elective SET in patients with a good prognosis is the only way at present to prevent many multiple births and associated adverse health outcomes.

PERINATAL OUTCOME IN SINGLETONS

A higher rate of preterm birth and LBW in IVF singleton pregnancies was found as early as 1985 in a study conducted in Australia[20]. A three-fold increase in the incidence of preterm birth in IVF singletons (19%) as compared with the general population was found.

Subsequently, several studies have described increased rates of preterm birth, LBW and small for gestational age (SGA) infants in singletons born after IVF.

It is well known from numerous publications that maternal characteristics in the ART population are different from those of the general population, e.g. higher maternal age, lower parity, duration of infertility and

underlying causes of infertility, which all are factors that may have a negative influence on outcome. In several studies, matching for one or more of
these variables has been performed. A summary of some of the matched
case–control studies is presented in Tables 4.2 and 4.3[21–28].

Koudstaal and co-workers performed the most elaborate matching for
an extensive number of maternal characteristics[27]. The proportion of
preterm birth, LBW and SGA was still significantly higher in the IVF
group. In cases with spontaneous onset of labor, gestational age at delivery
was 3 days shorter in the IVF group (275 vs. 278 days, $p = 0.05$). No difference was found in placental weight between the IVF and control
groups. The relatively LBW in association with normal placental weight
resulted in an increased placenta/birth weight ratio. According to the Barker hypothesis, these infants are possibly at risk of cardiovascular and other
diseases later in life. This correlation is, however, still controversial[29,30].

In other population-based studies data from different national registries
have been used with varying adjustments for differences in maternal characteristics. In the Swedish registry study of all IVF deliveries in Sweden
between 1982 and 1995, a strongly increased risk of very short duration of
gestation and very low birth weight (VLBW) was found in the IVF singleton group, as compared with the general population (risk ratios 3.54, 95%
CI 2.90–4.32; and 4.39, 95% CI 3.63–5.32, respectively)[12]. After stratification for maternal characteristics (maternal age, parity and duration of
infertility) the risk ratios decreased, but a small albeit significantly
increased risk remained (risk ratios 1.46, 95% CI 1.10–1.95 and 1.54, 95%
CI 1.17–2.03, respectively). In the Finnish registry study, Gissler et al. also
found increased risks of preterm birth and LBW after adjustment for
maternal background variables (county, smoking, age, marital status, previous pregnancies and previous deliveries): preterm birth < 37 weeks, OR
2.24, 95% CI 1.77–2.83 and LBW < 2500 g, OR 2.41, 95% CI 1.86–3.14[10].

In another large registry study performed in the USA, Schieve et al.
found an increased risk of LBW and VLBW in IVF singletons, as compared
with the general population (risk ratio 1.8, 95% CI 1.7–1.9 and 1.8, 95%
CI 1.7–2.0, respectively, after adjustment for maternal age and parity).
Increased risks were observed for all infertility diagnosis subsets, including
subgroups with presumably healthy gametes (oocytes from an egg donor
and sperm from a partner without a diagnosis of male factor infertility)[31].

Three meta-analyses have now been published concerning the perinatal outcome of singletons after assisted conception. Helmerhorst et al.
included 14 matched and three non-matched studies[32] and Jackson and co-
workers included 15 studies, both cohort studies and matched control
studies comprising 12 283 IVF and 1.9 million spontaneous conceptions[33].
The most recent meta-analysis performed by McDonald and co-workers

Table 4.2 Results of matched case–control studies in which *in vitro* fertilization (IVF) singleton pregnancies are compared with spontaneously conceived singleton pregnancies: preterm birth

| Author | Year of publication | Country | Preterm birth <37 weeks | | | Preterm birth <32 weeks | | |
			IVF (n, %)	Control (n, %)	RR or OR (CI) or p value	IVF (n, %)	Control (n, %)	RR or OR (CI) or p value
Tan[21]	1992	UK	69/494 (14)	78/978[a] (8)	1.78 (1.30–2.42)	NA	NA	
Tanbo[22]	1995	Norway	53/355[f] (14.9)	61/643[b] (9.5)	<0.01	NA	NA	
Verlaenen[23]	1995	Belgium	16/140 (11.4)	2/140[c] (1.4)	<0.01	NA	NA	
Reubinoff[24]	1997	Israel	23/260 (8.8)	10/260[d] (3.8)	0.024	NA	NA	
Dhont[25]	1997	Belgium	26/311 (8.4)	65/622[d] (10.5)	0.80 (0.52–1.23)	4/311 (1.3)	18/622 (2.9)	0.44 (0.15–1.30)
Dhont[26]	1999	Belgium	344/3048 (11.3)	125/3048[e] (4.1)	2.75 (2.26–3.36)	63/3048 (2.1)	8/3048 (0.3)	7.88 (3.78–16.4)

continued

66

Table 4.2 Continued

Author	Year of publication	Country	Preterm birth <37 weeks				Preterm birth <32 weeks			
			IVF (n, %)	Control (n, %)	RR or OR (CI) or p value		IVF (n, %)	Control (n, %)	RR or OR(CI) or p value	
Koudstaal[27]	2000	The Netherlands	46/307 (15.0)	18/307[f] (5.9)	0.001		NA	NA		
Koivurova[28]	2002	Finland	13/153 (8.5)	16/287[g] (5.6)	1.52 (0.75–3.08)		3/153 (2.0)	3/287 (1.0)	1.88 (0.38–9.18)	

RR, relative risk; OR, odds ratio; CI, confidence interval; NA, not available; [*]281 IVF, 23 gamete intra-Fallopian transfer (GIFT), 51 other artificial reproduction techniques. [a]Primiparous women, stratum matched for maternal age; [b]matched for maternal age, parity, same university hospital; [c]matched for maternal age, parity, height, weight, date of delivery, same university hospital; [d]matched for maternal age, parity, ethnic origin, location and date of delivery, same university hospital; [e]matched for maternal age, parity, fetal sex, date of delivery, same university hospital; [f]matched for maternal age, parity, ethnic origin, height, weight, smoking habits, date of delivery, medical disorders, obstetric history, obstetric department; [g]matched for sex, year of birth, area of residence, parity, maternal age, social class

Table 4.3 Results of matched case–control studies in which *in vitro* fertilization (IVF) singleton pregnancies are compared with spontaneously conceived singleton pregnancies: low birth weight

Author	Year of publication	Country	Low birth weight <2500 g			Very low birth weight <1500 g		
			IVF (n, %)	Control (n, %)	RR or OR (CI) or p value	IVF (n, %)	Control (n, %)	RR or OR (CI) or p value
Tan[21]	1992	UK	69/494 (14.0)	68/978[a] (6.9)	2.01 (1.46–2.76)	NA	NA	NA
Tanbo[22]	1995	Norway	41/355* (11.5)	43/643[b] (6.7)	1.73 (1.15–2.60)	14/355 (3.9)	15/643 (2.3)	1.69 (0.83–3.46)
Verlaenen[23]	1995	Belgium	14/140 (10.0)	6/140[c] (4.3)	2.33 (0.92–5.90)	5/140 (3.6)	1/140 (0.7)	5.00 (0.59–42.3)
Reubinoff[24]	1997	Israel	29/260 (11.2)	30/260[d] (11.6)	1.0	NA	NA	
Dhont[25]	1997	Belgium	24/311 (7.7)	70/622[e] (11.3)	0.69 (0.44–1.07)	5/311 (1.6)	17/622 (2.7)	0.59 (0.22–1.58)
Dhont[26]	1999	Belgium	319/3048 (10.5)	162/3048[e] (4.2)	1.97 (1.64–2.36)	72/3048 (2.4)	10/3048 (0.3)	7.20 (3.72–13.9)

continued

Table 4.3 *Continued*

Author	Year of publication	Country	Low birth weight < 2500 g			Very low birth weight < 1500 g		
			IVF (n, %)	Control (n, %)	RR or OR (CI) or p value	IVF (n, %)	Control (n, %)	RR or OR (CI) or p value
Koudstaal[27]	2000	The Netherlands	42/307 (13.7)	21/307[f] (6.8)	0.005	NA	NA	
Koivurova[28]	2002	Finland	9/153 (5.9)	9/287[g] (3.1)	1.88 (0.76–4.63)	3/153 (2.0)	2/287 (0.7)	2.81 (0.48–16.7)

[e]281 IVF, 23 gamete intra-Fallopian transfer (GIFT), 51 other artificial reproduction techniques. [a–g]see Table 4.2

included case–control studies, matched for at least maternal age[34]. A summary of the three meta-analyses is shown in Table 4.4. There is remarkable consistency both within each meta-analysis and between the meta-analyses. For example, IVF singleton pregnancies have adverse outcomes as compared with spontaneous conception, the risk of prematurity, LBW and perinatal mortality being about two-fold. Jackson and co-workers[33] also included some secondary outcomes in their meta-analysis. They showed that IVF singletons had increased ORs for stillbirth, spontaneous preterm birth, gestational diabetes, pre-eclampsia, placenta previa, vaginal bleeding, labor induction, elective and emergency cesarean section. However, the authors stated that these results should be interpreted with caution since they did not specifically search for studies with these outcomes, and for some outcomes the definitions varied from study to study.

Finally, two large cohort studies with comparable results, not included in the meta-analyses, from Australia and Sweden, have just been published. The Australian study, comprising more than 17 000 infants, showed an observed number of preterm births in singletons that was 2.4 times higher than the expected number in the general population and the observed number of LBW infants was 2.1 times higher than expected[35]. Singletons born to couples with female factor infertility were more likely to be born preterm and have LBW than singletons born to couples with male-factor infertility. The increased risk in IVF singletons persisted even when IVF singletons conceived with the transfer of only one embryo when compared with the general population. Otherwise, a better obstetric outcome might be expected for singletons after SET. In a recent Belgian study, SET singletons were found to compare favorably with spontaneously conceived singletons[36].

In a more recent study, further data for 1996–2001 were added to the Swedish registry study. The new analysis included 10 088 singleton births[37]. Absolute risks are given in this study, which may be more useful than relative risks in counseling patients. Preterm birth (<37 completed weeks) occurred in 9.6% as compared with 5.3% among all singleton births, and very preterm birth before 32 weeks occurred in 1.9% of the singleton infants born after IVF as compared with 0.7% among all singleton births. The corresponding figures for LBW and VLBW were 7.3% versus 3.5% and 1.8% versus 0.6% for IVF and control population, respectively. SGA occurred in 5.1% in IVF singletons and in 2.8% among all births.

In summary, there is a body of research related to perinatal outcome among IVF singletons showing that they are at increased risk of LBW, VLBW, preterm delivery and being born as SGA infants in comparison with spontaneously conceived singletons. The effect is larger for very preterm births than for mildly preterm births and for VLBW than for

Table 4.4 Results of meta-analyses of perinatal outcome in *in vitro* fertilization (IVF) singletons

	Helmerhorst et al., 2004[32]	Jackson et al., 2004[33]	McDonald et al., 2005[34]
Inclusion criteria	14 case–control studies	15 case–control studies and cohort studies	14 case–control studies
Sample size	5361 IVF and 7038 controls	12 283 IVF and 1.9 million controls	6728 IVF and 8454 controls
Outcomes			
Perinatal mortality	1.68 (1.11–2.55)*	2.2 (1.6–3.0)	2.40 (1.59–3.63)
Preterm birth, <37 weeks	2.04 (1.80–2.32)*	2.0 (1.7–2.2)	1.93 (1.36–2.74)
Very preterm birth, <32–33 weeks	3.27 (2.03–5.28)*	3.10 (2.00–4.80)	2.99 (1.54–5.80)
Low birth weight, <2500 g	1.70 (1.50–1.92)*	1.8 (1.4–2.2)	1.40 (1.01–1.95)
Very low birth weight, <1500 g	3.00 (2.07–4.36)*	2.7 (2.3–3.1)	3.78 (4.29–5.75)
Small for gestational age	1.40 (1.15–1.71)*	1.6 (1.3–2.0)	1.59 (1.20–2.11)
Cesarean section	1.54 (1.44–1.66)*	2.13 (1.72–2.63)	1.81 (1.41–2.32)
NICU	1.27 (1.16–1.40)*	1.60 (1.30–1.96)	1.36 (1.20–1.54)

NICU, neonatal intensive care unit. *Summary relative risk with 95% CI. The other figures are for summary odds ratio with 95% CI

LBW. However, it still remains unclear whether the increased risk of adverse outcome in IVF singletons is a direct effect of the IVF procedure, is a direct effect of components of the IVF procedure, or reflects some other factor related to the underlying infertility of the couple. Some studies suggest a treatment effect. In one of these studies singleton infants conceived with infertility treatment had a two-fold increase in LBW compared with infants conceived 3 or more months after infertility treatment was discontinued[38]. Other studies have suggested that infertility *per se* unrelated to treatment is associated with an increased risk of adverse obstetric outcome[39–41]. Altered management of IVF pregnancies may also give rise to bias, since both patients and doctors monitor IVF pregnancies more closely, which may lead to more hospitalizations and obstetric interventions. Induced labor and elective cesarean section are reported as more common interventions in IVF pregnancies than in spontaneous pregnancies, although it is likely that this would have a greater influence on outcomes such as moderate preterm birth than very preterm birth. In most studies it is not possible to distinguish preterm births owing to obstetric intervention from spontaneous preterm births. However, in some studies spontaneous preterm births were analyzed[21,23,24,27], and when included in the meta-analyses by Jackson *et al.*, the summary ORs for spontaneous preterm births were indeed increased in IVF pregnancies[33]. Although it is not feasible to perform the most accurate study, which would be a randomized controlled trial, there is a need for other well-designed studies to further evaluate and distinguish treatment effects from infertility effects.

PERINATAL OUTCOME IN TWINS

Twin pregnancies are divided into two major types: dizygotic (DZ) and monozygotic (MZ) twin pregnancies. The rate of MZ twinning in the general population is believed to be fairly constant around the world and over time (3–4 per 1000 pregnancies). The incidence of DZ twinning in the population is affected by many factors such as race, heredity, maternal age, and ovulation induction, and is more variable, ranging from 3 to 40 per 1000 pregnancies[42,43]. In Caucasians about 30% of twin pregnancies are MZ and about 70% are DZ.

There are two major types of placenta: monochorionic (MC) and dichorionic (DC), depending on the histologic composition of the dividing membrane. In MC placentas, the septum consists of two layers of amnion, while in DC placentas it has two layers of amnion and two layers of chorion. If the dividing membrane is absent, the condition is described as a monoamniotic (MA), MC twin gestation. DC placentas are found in about 80% of twin gestations and can be associated with either DZ or MZ twins. DC placentas may be separate or fused. MC placentation, which may be either MA or diamniotic (DA), accounts for 20% of twin gestations and is present only in MZ twins.

Although most of the multiple gestations following ART appear to be DZ, i.e. the fertilization of two ova by different spermatozoa (due to dual embryo transfer), MZ twinning, from embryo splitting, is also of concern. In 1987, Derom *et al.* noted a two-fold increase in the MZ rate among pregnancies as the result of ovulation-inducing medications, most without ART[44]. Subsequent reports documented higher rates of MZ twinning (from 1% to 5%) among pregnancies after ART than typically observed in the population[45-50]. Two specific treatment factors in ART appear to be particularly risky: assisted hatching (use of chemicals, lasers, or mechanical means to create an opening in the embryo's zona pellucida) and blastocyst (or extended) culture.

Recent studies have shown that it is chorionicity rather than zygosity that determines outcome in twin gestations, with MC twins being at higher risk of adverse outcome than DC twins[51]. In twin studies, consideration must therefore be taken of variations and type of zygosity in different populations.

A more adverse outcome in IVF twins, as compared with twins after spontaneous conception, might be expected owing to maternal background characteristics, resembling the situation for IVF singleton pregnancies. However, the higher rate of MZ twinning in spontaneous twins, as compared with IVF twins (30% vs. 1–5%), may influence outcome, i.e. IVF twins should be expected to have better outcomes than spontaneously conceived twins.

Two recent meta-analyses of perinatal outcomes in IVF twins have been published (Table 4.5). In the meta-analysis by Helmerhorst and co-workers, nine matched studies comprising 3437 IVF/ICSI twins and 3429 control twins were analyzed[32]. The relative risk (RR) of preterm birth was 1.07 (95% CI 1.02–1.13) and the RR of very preterm birth was 0.95 (95% CI 0.78–1.15) in matched studies. Preterm twins differed widely in frequency: 18.8–60.0% and 20.0–52.4% in IVF and control group, respectively. The RR for LBW and VLBW in the matched studies was 1.03 (95% CI 0.99–1.08) and 0.89 (95% CI 0.74–1.07). No difference was seen for SGA rates in IVF and spontaneous twins. Rates of cesarean section and admissions to neonatal intensive care units (NICUs) were significantly higher after assisted conception than after spontaneous conception.

Table 4.5 Results of meta-analyses of perinatal outcome in *in vitro* fertilization (IVF) twins

	Helmerhorst *et al.*, 2004[32]	McDonald *et al.*, 2005[53]
Inclusion criteria	10 case–control studies	8 case–control studies
Sample size	3437 IVF twins, 3429 spontaneously conceived twins	2303 IVF twins, 2326 spontaneously conceived twins
Outcomes		
Perinatal mortality	0.58 (0.44–0.77)*	1.40 (0.22–9.11)
Preterm birth, <37 weeks	1.07 (1.02–1.13)*	1.41 (0.96–2.08)[†] 1.57 (1.01–2.44)[††] week 32–36: 1.48 (1.05–2.10)
Very preterm birth, <32–33 weeks	0.95 (0.78–1.15)*	1.03 (0.4–2.9)
Low birth weight, <2500 g	1.03 (0.99–1.08)*	1.13 (0.85–1.51)
Very low birth weight, <1500 g	0.89 (0.74–1.07)*	1.22 (0.5–2.9)
Small for gestational age	1.27 (0.97–1.65)*	0.92 (0.62–1.38)
Cesarean section	1.21 (1.11–1.32)*	1.33 (1.06–1.67)
NICU	1.05 (1.01–1.09)*	2.22 (1.64–3.02)

NICU, neonatal intensive care unit. *Summary relative risk and 95% CI. The other figures are for summary odds ratio and 95% CI. [†]Matched at least for maternal age; [††]controlled for maternal age and parity

Nevertheless, IVF twins had lower perinatal mortality than spontaneous twins (RR 0.58, 95% CI 0.44–0.77). However, it should be mentioned that in one of the studies included, the control group had very high perinatal mortality (48/216 = 222/1000) compared with the IVF group (4/112 = 35.7/1000)[52].

The other meta-analysis, by McDonald and co-workers, included 11 case–control studies comprising 2303 IVF twins and 2326 spontaneously conceived twins[53]. There were some differences in methods between the two analyses but the results were very similar. Compared with spontaneously conceived twins, when matched for maternal age, IVF twins were at increased risk of preterm birth between 32 and 37 weeks of gestation (OR 1.48, 95% CI 1.05–2.10) and had an elevated risk of preterm birth at < 37 weeks of gestation (OR 1.57, 95% CI 1.01–2.44) when also matched for parity. IVF twins were also more likely to be delivered by cesarean section (OR 1.33, 95% CI 1.06–1.67). No differences were seen in incidence of perinatal death, SGA or LBW infants. The authors' conclusion was that IVF twins have adverse perinatal outcome as compared with spontaneous twins, but the differences are much smaller than between IVF singletons and spontaneous singletons. One speculation is that in a low-risk singleton pregnancy an added risk such as assisted conception may have a marked impact, while it may have only a small impact on a high-risk twin pregnancy.

Four large Nordic cohort studies have been published but were not included in these meta-analyses. The Swedish[12] and Norwegian studies[54] showed no difference in perinatal mortality but an increased rate of cesarean deliveries among IVF twins as compared with other twins. The Finnish study[55] showed a higher rate of LBW infants even after adjustment for maternal background factors. In the Danish study, Pinborg et al. found no difference in preterm birth, very preterm birth, LBW or VLBW between IVF/ICSI twins and spontaneous twins[56]. The same results were found when only different-sex twins (i.e. only DZ twins) were compared[56]. A comprehensive overview of short- and long-term consequences of IVF/ICSI twins is presented in a recent review[57].

In conclusion, the existing literature has shown that IVF twins may have slightly worse perinatal outcomes than twins conceived spontaneously, despite the fact that their outcomes should be better because of the decreased proportion of MC twins in IVF pregnancies. The adverse effect in IVF twins is much less than in IVF singletons. However, in comparison with IVF singletons, IVF twins fare noticeably worse in terms of virtually all perinatal morbidities.

PERINATAL OUTCOME IN TRIPLETS AND HIGHER-ORDER MULTIPLE BIRTHS

Since the introduction of assisted conception in the latest decades the incidence of triplets and high-order multiple births has risen dramatically in many countries around the world. Numerous studies have documented increased obstetric and neonatal complications in triplet and higher-order pregnancies compared with twins or singletons. However, very little information is available from controlled studies concerning the outcome in triplets and higher-order multiple births after IVF. Seoud et al.[58] studied perinatal outcome in 115 twin, 15 triplet and four quadruplet IVF pregnancies from one IVF program and found a proportionate progressive increase in obstetric and neonatal complications for twins, triplets and quadruplets. Roest et al.[59] compared 23 sets of triplets and one set of quadruplets after IVF with 54 sets of IVF twins, showing that triplets and higher-order infants were born at a lower gestational age, had lower birth weights and higher rates of longer-duration hospital admissions than twins. In addition to the more adverse obstetric outcome, there are more psychological and social complications associated with triplet and higher-order births[60,61]. The need to minimize triplet and higher-order pregnancies following assisted conception is obvious.

PERINATAL OUTCOME IN ICSI PREGNANCIES

Since the introduction of ICSI there have been many safety concerns, as ICSI is a more invasive procedure than conventional IVF. The ICSI technique gives infertile couples the possibility of achieving a biological pregnancy, which would otherwise have been impossible. Concerns about the safety of ICSI are related to the ICSI technique itself and to the use of sperm that may carry chromosomal and genetic abnormalities.

Bonduelle et al. have carried out the largest prospective, controlled study to date comparing pregnancies conceived after conventional IVF with those conceived after ICSI. In their most recent analysis, they reported on a cohort of 2889 infants born after ICSI and 2995 infants born after IVF. ICSI was performed using ejaculated, epididymal and testicular sperm[62]. The results are presented in Table 4.6. The prematurity rate was slightly higher in the ICSI than in the IVF group, reflecting a higher prematurity rate in ICSI multiples. Birth weight, LBW, perinatal death and neonatal complications were similar for the ICSI and IVF groups. Other authors, such as Govaerts et al.[63], did not find a higher prematurity rate in ICSI twins, as compared with IVF twins, and Wennerholm et al.[64] and Loft

Table 4.6 Results of a prospective study comparing infants born after intra-cytoplasmic sperm injection (ICSI) with those born after conventional *in vitro* fertilization (IVF). Adapted from reference 62

Outcome parameter	ICSI	IVF	p Value
Infants (n)	2889	2995	
Preterm birth, <37 weeks (%)			
all	31.8	29.3	0.046
singletons	8.4 (n = 1499)	9.0 (n = 1556)	
twins	54.6 (n = 1228)	47.6 (n = 1250)	
triplets	94.7 (n = 113)	NA	
Birth weight (g)			
all, mean	2807	2765	0.060
singletons, mean	3224 (n = 1499)	3176 (n = 1556)	
twins, mean	2394 (n = 1228)	2382 (n = 1250)	
triplets, mean	1762 (n = 113)	1769 (n = 145)	
LBW, <2500 g (%)			
all	26.7	26.5	0.858
singletons	7.1 (n = 1499)	7.8 (n = 1556)	
twins	48.1 (n = 1228)	45.1 (n = 1250)	
triplets	54.0 (n = 113)	NA	
VLBW, <1500 g (%)			
all	4.4	5.6	0.031
singletons	1.5 (n = 1499)	1.8 (n = 1556)	
twins	5.2 (n = 1228)	7.6 (n = 1250)	
triplets	34.5 (n = 113)	NA	
PNM, ≥20 weeks (%)			
all	1.87	2.33	0.238
singletons	1.25 (n = 1499)	0.77 (n = 1556)	
twins	2.38 (n = 1228)	3.87 (n = 1250)	
triplets	4.27 (n = 113)	NA	

NA, not available; LBW, low birth weight; VLBW, very low birth weight; PNM, perinatal mortality

et al.[65] reported lower prematurity rates in ICSI twins in their studies (42.3% and 35%, respectively); however, without any control groups. ICSI singletons had similar prematurity rates as IVF singletons.

In a prospective German study, pregnancies resulting from ejaculated sperm, testicular biopsies and epididymal aspirates were recruited before the 16th week of gestation and analyzed regarding pregnancy outcome and birth data, including malformations[66]. These researchers found no risk associated with the use of epididymal or testicular sperm, compared with ejaculated sperm, and the number of sperm in the ejaculate did not influence results. In the latest Swedish registry study, comprising 16 280 infants (4955 ICSI infants) comparisons were made between conventional IVF and ICSI singleton births. No significant difference was seen in the risk for preterm birth, LBW and low Apgar score after adjustments for year of birth, maternal age, parity, smoking and years of involuntary childlessness[37]. Similar results were shown in another large Belgian study[67].

In conclusion, ICSI does not seem to have any negative influence on perinatal outcome, and the results are comparable to those with conventional IVF.

PERINATAL OUTCOME AFTER CRYOPRESERVATION OF EMBRYOS

Cryopreservation of embryos is well established in most IVF programs today. With a strategy of transferring fewer embryos there will be an increase in the number of embryos available for cryopreservation, and there will be more pregnancies after replacement of frozen–thawed embryos. Frozen–thawed embryos are predominantly replaced in a natural cycle without the use of superovulation, which might influence perinatal outcome positively. However, concerns were raised 11 years ago when a study performed on adult mice born after cryopreservation showed morphological and behavioral disorders[68].

There have been surprisingly few studies addressing the outcome of children born after cryopreservation. In the Swedish national IVF cohort, singletons born after cryopreservation had a significantly lower risk of preterm birth and LBW when compared with conventional IVF in a stimulated cycle[12]. In the latest Swedish registry study, more than 1000 infants born after cryopreservation were compared with more than 10 000 infants born after conventional IVF. Significantly lower ORs were found for preterm birth (OR 0.69, 95% CI 0.58–0.83), LBW (OR 0.49, 95% CI 0.02–0.75) and low Apgar score (OR 0.26, 95% CI 0.09–0.78)[37]. In another Swedish case–control study, there was also a tendency toward a better outcome in the cryopreservervation group, as compared with the conventional IVF group, but this difference was not significant[69]. Most studies show similar results for IVF cycles using fresh or cryopreserved embryos and there is, to our knowledge, no study that indicates a negative effect on perinatal outcome in pregnancies after cryopreservation[70–75].

PERINATAL OUTCOME AFTER OVUM DONATION

Ovum donation was introduced 20 years ago as a treatment for infertility. The main indications for ovum donation IVF are premature ovarian failure or dysfunction, previously failed multiple IVF attempts and women carrying transmittable genetic abnormalities that could affect offspring. There is only limited literature addressing specific risks with these pregnancies. Most of the studies published on obstetric outcome after ovum donation have shown a significant increase in pregnancy-induced hypertension and pre-eclampsia, reported in 23–38% of the pregnancies[76–79]. This has been attributable to advanced maternal age and to the fact that these pregnancies are immunologically alien to the recipient. Other obstetric complications, which have been reported to occur in excess in egg-donation pregnancies, are an increased incidence of SGA infants and a higher risk of postpartum hemorrhage[76]. However, most of these studies have not had appropriate comparison groups. In a recent retrospective analysis, egg-donation pregnancies were compared with conventional IVF pregnancies. Obstetric outcome was good and did not differ between the two groups, with the exception of pregnancy-induced hypertension[79]. The limitations of that study were, as in many of the other studies, the relatively small sample size.

NEONATAL MORBIDITY

The high rate of multiple births and the increased risk of prematurity and LBW in both singletons and multiples will affect the risk of severe neonatal complications among infants born. Meta-analyses have shown increased NICU admissions in both IVF singletons[32,33] and IVF twins[32,53] as compared with controls. Increased neonatal hospitalization for IVF children was also found by Ericson et al. and Klemetti et al.[80,81]. Pinborg et al. also found an increased risk for IVF twins being admitted to the NICU as compared with both spontaneous twins[56] and IVF/ICSI singletons[82]. Studies that suggest that IVF children are at increased risk of various adverse neonatal outcomes[37,81,83] have mainly not sufficiently addressed whether these risks were independent of LBW, preterm birth or multiple birth or were an effect of one of these. Källen and co-workers studied low Apgar scores and certain neonatal diagnoses, e.g. cerebral hemorrhage, convulsions, respiratory problems and sepsis, using the Swedish Medical Birth register as well as the Hospital Discharge Register[37]. Low Apgar score, < 7 at 5 min, was found in 2.6% of the IVF infants as compared with 1.3% in the general population. In IVF singletons, 1.8% had low Apgar scores, as compared with 1.3% in the general population; the OR adjusted for year of birth was 1.29 (95% CI 1.11–1.50). Higher rates of cerebral hemorrhage, neonatal convulsions, respiratory problems including mechanical ventilation or constant positive airway pressure (CPAP) and neonatal sepsis were also seen. These were mainly effects of the high rate of multiple births. In one case–control study of intraventricular hemorrhage, cases of intraventricular hemorrhage and controls were closely matched for both gestational age and birth weight and included equivalent proportions of multiples[83]. Adjusted OR was four-fold and statistically significant for the association between fertility treatment (mainly IVF) and intraventricular hemorrhage. However, this finding needs to be confirmed in further studies.

CONCLUSIONS

Most of the children born after IVF have favorable perinatal outcomes. The single most important impact of assisted conception on the perinatal outcome remains high multiple pregnancy rates. Fetuses in multiple pregnancies face much greater problems than singletons during pregnancy, delivery and in the neonatal period. Twins, regarded by some as an acceptable outcome of assisted conception, are also at increased risk of developing perinatal problems as compared with singletons. One obvious way of reducing the number of multiple pregnancies is to limit the number of transferred embryos to one embryo per cycle in all patients or in a selected group of patients.

However, elimination of multiple pregnancies will not totally eliminate the risks associated with IVF pregnancies, since there is a body of evidence demonstrating that among IVF singletons there is also an as yet unexplained increased risk of adverse perinatal outcome as compared with spontaneous singletons, even when adjusted for maternal characteristics. Further research should be conducted to address these questions and, if possible, improve treatments, in the hope of decreasing the risk for some outcomes.

REFERENCES

1. Steptoe PC, Edwards RG. Birth after the reimplantation of a human embryo. Lancet 1978; 2: 366
2. Bergh C. Single embryo transfer: a mini-review. Hum Reprod 2005; 20: 323–7

3. Andersen-Nyboe A, Gianaroli L, Felberbaum R, et al. Assisted reproductive technology in Europe, 2001. Results generated from European registers by ESHRE. Hum Reprod 2005; 20: 1158–76

4. Westmore A. First freeze–thaw baby is born. Australia pioneers the freeze–thaw embryo. New Sci 1984; 102: 3

5. Palermo G, Joris H, Devroey P, Van Steirteghem AC. Pregnancies after intracytoplasmic injection of single spermatozoon into an oocyte. Lancet 1992; 340: 17–18

6. Wright VC, Schieve LA, Reynolds MA, et al. Assisted reproductive technology surveillance – United States, 2001. MMWR Surveill Summ 2004; 53: 1–20

7. Kissin DM, Schieve LA, Reynolds MA. Multiple-birth risk associated with IVF and extended embryo culture: USA, 2001. Hum Reprod 2005; 20: 2215–23

8. MRC. Births in Great Britain resulting from assisted conception, 1978–87. MRC Working Party on Children Conceived by In Vitro Fertilisation. Br Med J 1990; 300: 1229–33

9. Friedler S, Mashiach S, Laufer N. Births in Israel resulting from in-vitro fertilization/embryo transfer, 1982–1989: National Registry of the Israeli Association for Fertility Research. Hum Reprod 1992; 7: 1159–63

10. Gissler M, Malin Silverio M, Hemminki E. In-vitro fertilization pregnancies and perinatal health in Finland 1991–1993. Hum Reprod 1995; 10: 1856–61

11. Rufat P, Olivennes F, de Mouzon J, et al. Task force report on the outcome of pregnancies and children conceived by in vitro fertilization (France: 1987 to 1989). Fertil Steril 1994; 61: 324–30

12. Bergh T, Ericson A, Hillensjo T, et al. Deliveries and children born after in-vitro fertilisation in Sweden 1982–95: a retrospective cohort study. Lancet 1999; 354: 1579–85

13. Dare MR, Crowther CA, Dodd JM, Norman RJ. Single or multiple embryo transfer following in vitro fertilisation for improved neonatal outcome: a systematic review of the literature. Aust NZ J Obstet Gynaecol 2004; 44: 283–91

14. Kallen B, Finnstrom O, Nygren KG, Olausson PO. Temporal trends in multiple births after in vitro fertilisation in Sweden, 1982–2001: a register study. Br Med J 2005; 331: 382–3

15. Thurin A, Hausken J, Hillensjo T, et al. Elective single-embryo transfer versus double-embryo transfer in in vitro fertilization. N Engl J Med 2004; 351: 2392–402

16. Kjellberg AT, Carlsson P, Bergh C. Randomized single versus double embryo transfer: obstetric and paediatric outcome and a cost-effectiveness analysis. Hum Reprod 2006; 21: 210–16

17. Gerris J, De Sutter P, De Neubourg D, et al. A real-life prospective health economic study of elective single embryo transfer versus two-embryo transfer in first IVF/ICSI cycles. Hum Reprod 2004; 19: 917–23

18. Pandian Z, Templeton A, Serour G, Bhattacharya S. Number of embryos for transfer after IVF and ICSI: a Cochrane review. Hum Reprod 2005; 20: 2681–7

19. Bergh C, Thurin-Kjellberg A, Karlström PO. Single embryo fertilization in vitro. Maintained birth rate in spite of dramatically reduced multiple birth frequency [In Swedish]. Lakartidningen 2005; 102: 3444–7, 3449

20. Lancaster PA. Obstetric outcome. Clin Obstet Gynaecol 1985; 12: 847–64

21. Tan SL, Doyle P, Campbell S, et al. Obstetric outcome of in vitro fertilization pregnancies compared with normally conceived pregnancies. Am J Obstet Gynecol 1992; 167: 778–84

22. Tanbo T, Dale PO, Lunde O, et al. Obstetric outcome in singleton pregnancies after assisted reproduction. Obstet Gynecol 1995; 86: 188–92

23. Verlaenen H, Cammu H, Derde MP, Amy JJ. Singleton pregnancy after in vitro fertilization: expectations and outcome. Obstet Gynecol 1995; 86: 906–10

24. Reubinoff BE, Samueloff A, Ben-Haim M, et al. Is the obstetric outcome of in vitro fertilized singleton gestations different from natural ones? A controlled study. Fertil Steril 1997; 67: 1077–83

25. Dhont M, De Neubourg F, Van der Elst J, De Sutter P. Perinatal outcome of pregnancies after assisted reproduction: a case–control study. J Assist Reprod Genet 1997; 14: 575–80

26. Dhont M, De Sutter P, Ruyssinck G, et al. Perinatal outcome of pregnancies after assisted reproduction: a case–control study. Am J Obstet Gynecol 1999; 181: 688–95

27. Koudstaal J, Braat DD, Bruinse HW, et al. Obstetric outcome of singleton pregnancies after IVF: a matched control study in four Dutch university hospitals. Hum Reprod 2000; 15: 1819–25

28. Koivurova S, Hartikainen AL, Gissler M, et al. Neonatal outcome and congenital malformations in children born after in-vitro fertilization. Hum Reprod 2002; 17: 1391–8

29. Barker DJ. In utero programming of cardiovascular disease. Theriogenology 2000; 53: 555–74

30. Barker DJ, Bull AR, Osmond C, Simmonds SJ. Fetal and placental size and risk of hypertension in adult life. Br Med J 1990; 301: 259–62

31. Schieve LA, Meikle SF, Ferre C, et al. Low and very low birth weight in infants conceived with use of assisted reproductive technology. N Engl J Med 2002; 346: 731–7

32. Helmerhorst FM, Perquin DA, Donker D, Keirse MJ. Perinatal outcome of singletons and twins after assisted conception: a systematic review of controlled studies. Br Med J 2004; 328: 261

33. Jackson RA, Gibson KA, Wu YW, Croughan MS. Perinatal outcomes in singletons following in vitro fertilization: a meta-analysis. Obstet Gynecol 2004; 103: 551–63

34. McDonald SD, Murphy K, Beyene J, Ohlsson A. Perinatal outcomes of singleton pregnancies achieved by in vitro fertilization: a systematic review and meta-analysis. J Obstet Gynaecol Can 2005; 27: 449–59

35. Wang YA, Sullivan EA, Black D, et al. Preterm birth and low birth weight after assisted reproductive technology-related pregnancy in Australia between 1996 and 2000. Fertil Steril 2005; 83: 1650–8

36. De Neubourg D, Mangelshots K, Van Royen E, et al. The obstetric and neonatal outcome of babies born after single embryo transfer in IVF/ICSI does not

compare unfavourably to spontaneously conceived babies. Hum Reprod 2005; 20 (Suppl 1): O–151

37. Kallen B, Finnstrom O, Nygren KG, Olausson PO. In vitro fertilization (IVF) in Sweden: infant outcome after different IVF fertilization methods. Fertil Steril 2005; 84: 611–17

38. Sundstrom I, Ildgruben A, Hogberg U. Treatment-related and treatment-independent deliveries among infertile couples, a long-term follow-up. Acta Obstet Gynecol Scand 1997; 76: 238–43

39. Basso O, Baird DD. Infertility and preterm delivery, birthweight, and Caesarean section: a study within the Danish National Birth Cohort. Hum Reprod 2003; 18: 2478–84

40. Pandian Z, Bhattacharya S, Templeton A. Review of unexplained infertility and obstetric outcome: a 10 year review. Hum Reprod 2001; 16: 2593–7

41. Thomson F. Shanbhag S, Templeton A, Bhattacharya S. Obstetric outcome in women with subfertility. Br J Obstet Gynaecol 2005; 112: 632–7

42. Derom C, Derom R, Vlietinck R, et al. Iatrogenic multiple pregnancies in East Flanders, Belgium. Fertil Steril 1993; 60: 493–6

43. Derom R, Orlebeke J, Eriksson A, Thiery M. The epidemiology of multiple births in Europe. In: Keith LG, Papiernik E, Keith DM, Luke B, eds. Multiple Pregnancy, Epidemiology, Gestation and Perinatal Outcome. Carnforth, UK: Parthenon Publishing, 1995: 145–62

44. Derom C, Vlietinck R, Derom R, et al. Increased monozygotic twinning rate after ovulation induction. Lancet 1987; 1: 1236–8

45. Alikani M, Cekleniak NA, Walters E, Cohen J. Monozygotic twinning following assisted conception: an analysis of 81 consecutive cases. Hum Reprod 2003; 18: 1937–43

46. Elizur SE, Levron J, Shrim A, et al. Monozygotic twinning is not associated with zona pellucida micromanipulation procedures but increases with high-order multiple pregnancies. Fertil Steril 2004; 82: 500–1

47. Milki AA, Jun SH, Hinckley MD, et al. Incidence of monozygotic twinning with blastocyst transfer compared to cleavage-stage transfer. Fertil Steril 2003; 79: 503–6

48. Schachter M, Raziel A, Friedler S, et al. Monozygotic twinning after assisted reproductive techniques: a phenomenon independent of micromanipulation. Hum Reprod 2001; 16: 1264–9

49. Schieve LA, Meikle SF, Peterson HB, et al. Does assisted hatching pose a risk for monozygotic twinning in pregnancies conceived through in vitro fertilization? Fertil Steril 2000; 74: 288–94

50. Sills ES, Moomjy M, Zaninovic N, et al. Human zona pellucida micromanipulation and monozygotic twinning frequency after IVF. Hum Reprod 2000; 15: 890–5

51. Sebire NJ, Snijders RJ, Hughes K, et al. The hidden mortality of monochorionic twin pregnancies. Br J Obstet Gynaecol 1997; 104: 1203–7

52. Fitzsimmons BP, Bebbington MW, Fluker MR. Perinatal and neonatal outcomes in multiple gestations: assisted reproduction versus spontaneous conception. Am J Obstet Gynecol 1998; 179: 1162–7

53. McDonald S, Murphy K, Beyene J, Ohlsson A. Perinatal outcomes of in vitro fertilization twins: a systematic review and meta-analyses. Am J Obstet Gynecol 2005; 193: 141–52

54. von During V, Maltau JM, Forsdahl F, et al. [Pregnancy, births and infants after in-vitro fertilization in Norway, 1988–1991]. Tidsskr Nor Laegeforen 1995; 115: 2054–60

55. Gissler M, Hemminki E. The danger of overmatching in studies of the perinatal mortality and birthweight of infants born after assisted conception. Eur J Obstet Gynecol Reprod Biol 1996; 69: 73–5

56. Pinborg A, Loft A, Rasmussen S, et al. Neonatal outcome in a Danish national cohort of 3438 IVF/ICSI and 10362 non-IVF/ICSI twins born between 1995 and 2000. Hum Reprod 2004; 19: 435–41

57. Pinborg A. IVF/ICSI twin pregnancies: risks and prevention. Hum Reprod Update 2005; 11: 575–93

58. Seoud MA, Toner JP, Kruithoff C, Muasher SJ. Outcome of twin, triplet, and quadruplet in vitro fertilization pregnancies: the Norfolk experience. Fertil Steril 1992; 57: 825–34

59. Roest J, van Heusden AM, Verhoeff A, et al. A triplet pregnancy after in vitro fertilization is a procedure-related complication that should be prevented by replacement of two embryos only. Fertil Steril 1997; 67: 290–5

60. Garel M, Blondel B. Assessment at 1 year of the psychological consequences of having triplets. Hum Reprod 1992; 7: 729–32

61. Garel M, Salobir C, Blondel B. Psychological consequences of having triplets: a 4-year follow-up study. Fertil Steril 1997; 67: 1162–5

62. Bonduelle M, Liebaers I, Deketelaere V, et al. Neonatal data on a cohort of 2889 infants born after ICSI (1991–1999) and of 2995 infants born after IVF (1983–1999). Hum Reprod 2002: 17: 671–94

63. Govaerts I, Devreker F, Koenig I, et al. Comparison of pregnancy outcome after intracytoplasmic sperm injection and in-vitro fertilization. Hum Reprod 1998; 13: 1514–18

64. Wennerholm UB, Bergh C, Hamberger L, et al. Obstetric and perinatal outcome of pregnancies following intracytoplasmic sperm injection. Hum Reprod 1996; 11: 1113–19

65. Loft A, Petersen K, Erb K, et al. A Danish national cohort of 730 infants born after intracytoplasmic sperm injection (ICSI) 1994–1997. Hum Reprod 1999; 14: 2143–8

66. Ludwig M, Katalinic A. Pregnancy course and health of children born after ICSI depending on parameters of male factor infertility. Hum Reprod 2003; 18: 351–7

67. Ombelet W, Cadron I, Gerris J, et al. Obstetric and perinatal outcome of 1655 ICSI and 3974 IVF singleton and 1102 ICSI and 2901 IVF twin births: a comparative analysis. Reprod Biomed Online 2005; 11: 76–85

68. Dulioust E, Toyama K, Busnel MC, et al. Long-term effects of embryo freezing in mice. Proc Natl Acad Sci USA 1995; 92: 589–93
69. Wennerholm UB, Hamberger L, Nilsson L, et al. Obstetric and perinatal outcome of children conceived from cryopreserved embryos. Hum Reprod 1997; 12: 1819–25
70. Olivennes F, Schneider Z, Remy V, et al. Perinatal outcome and follow-up of 82 children aged 1–9 years old conceived from cryopreserved embryos. Hum Reprod 1996; 11: 1565–8
71. Sutcliffe AG. Follow-up of children conceived from cryopreserved embryos. Mol Cell Endocrinol 2000; 169: 91–3
72. Sutcliffe AG, D'Souza SW, Cadman J, et al. Outcome in children from cryopreserved embryos. Arch Dis Child 1995; 72: 290–3
73. Wada I, Macnamee MC, Wick K, et al. Birth characteristics and perinatal outcome of babies conceived from cryopreserved embryos. Hum Reprod 1994; 9: 543–6
74. Wennerholm UB, Albertsson-Wikland K, Bergh C, et al. Postnatal growth and health in children born after cryopreservation as embryos. Lancet 1998; 351: 1085–90
75. Wennerholm WB. Cryopreservation of embryos and oocytes: obstetric outcome and health in children. Hum Reprod 2000; 15 (Suppl 5): 18–25
76. Abdalla HI, Billett A, Kan AK, et al. Obstetric outcome in 232 ovum donation pregnancies. Br J Obstet Gynaecol 1998; 105: 332–7
77. Sheffer-Mimouni G, Mashiach S, Dor J, et al. Factors influencing the obstetric and perinatal outcome after oocyte donation. Hum Reprod 2002; 17: 2636–40
78. Soderstrom-Anttila V, Tiitinen A, Foudila T, Hovatta O. Obstetric and perinatal outcome after oocyte donation: comparison with in-vitro fertilization pregnancies. Hum Reprod 1998; 13: 483–90
79. Wiggins DA, Main E. Outcomes of pregnancies achieved by donor egg in vitro fertilization – a comparison with standard in vitro fertilization pregnancies. Am J Obstet Gynecol 2005; 192: 2002–6; discussion 2006–8
80. Ericson A, Nygren KG, Olausson PO, Kallen B. Hospital care utilization of infants born after IVF. Hum Reprod 2002; 17: 929–32
81. Klemetti R, Gissler M, Hemminki E. Comparison of perinatal health of children born from IVF in Finland in the early and late 1990s. Hum Reprod 2002; 17: 2192–8
82. Pinborg A, Loft A, Nyboe Andersen A. Neonatal outcome in a Danish national cohort of 8602 children born after in vitro fertilization or intracytoplasmic sperm injection: the role of twin pregnancy. Acta Obstet Gynecol Scand 2004; 83: 1071–8
83. Linder N, Haskin O, Levit O, et al. Risk factors for intraventricular hemorrhage in very low birth weight premature infants: a retrospective case–control study. Pediatrics 2003; 111: e590–5

Chapter 5

Neurodevelopmental and neurological outcome in children born after assisted reproductive therapies

Alastair G Sutcliffe

This chapter reviews the known literature regarding neurodevelopmental outcome after assisted reproductive technology (ART). What it will not do is refer to studies of twins or higher-order births because they will separately be referred to in the chapter written by Elizabeth Bryan and Jane Denton (Chapter 8).

Before reviewing the literature there are some basic concepts, which the reader needs to understand, about neurodevelopmental outcome studies. First and foremost intellectual development, which is tested in the child via a neurodevelopmental assessment, is one of the most important aspects of outcome for the health of any child. This is whether they are recovering from an illness or are born after an intrauterine intervention (i.e. 'fetal exposure') or indeed in the case of an ART-conceived child; they may be susceptible to neurodevelopmental problems by the nature of their conception (and periconceptual events/risks).

When a parent asks 'is my child going to be healthy, Doctor?' what underpins that question includes the all-important physical wellbeing and the equally important, possibly even more important, educational/ intellectual wellbeing. Thus studies which have been performed to answer these questions over the years are worthwhile. A reduction in neurodevelopmental attainment from any form of illness or events in the child's life, either due to an event in pregnancy, perinatally, in infancy, or later on in their life, can have profound effects not just on the child and their family but also on society as a whole (via an economic impact). For example, if 2% of ART children are neurodevelopmentally delayed against a population average of 1% then it is not hard to understand the potential economic impact.

Neurodevelopmental assessment of children is a science which is underpinned by psychological theory, psychometric methodology and skilled observer assessment. To the naive outsider observing the assessment of a young child may seem like play (Figure 5.1). But as Shakespeare says 'and thereby hangs a tale'. Indeed, the way that children, especially of a younger age, are communicated with, and show their knowledge/intellect, is via play. This is especially true in very young children who do not have formal language capacities that can be categorized in a similar manner to those of adults or older children.

The value of a neurodevelopmental assessment is that it reflects brain development and functioning, and ultimately intelligence. Although it must be remembered by the reader that it is currently thought by the best available evidence that two-thirds of intelligence is hereditary and one-third is as a result of environment/educational stimulation. The hereditary aspects of intelligence are no different in an ART-conceived child than in a naturally conceived child, except where there are donor gametes involved. Historically there has been a tendency for the ART-conceived child to be born to parents from higher socioeconomic status/background and thus potentially more likely to be intellectually advanced. This fact has confounded reported studies.

This leads on to the nature of neurodevelopmental studies and how they can potentially give misleading results. There are a number of

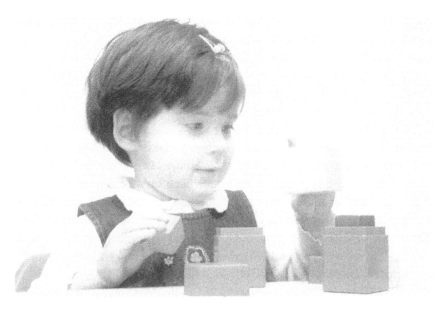

Figure 5.1 Performing one item of the Griffiths scales of mental development for children 0–2 years of age

potential ways in which assessments can be flawed. These can start with, for example, the observer of the child, who may not be applying the testing system with appropriate rigor and consistency. The child themself may be tired when being assessed and this could affect the representativeness of their assessment. The testing system being used may not have been recently standardized. Standardization is important because it has been shown consistently, regardless of the neurodevelopmental system being used (examples of which include Griffiths scales of mental development, Bayley scales of mental development, Weschler infant and primary school preschool scales of intelligence, etc.), that children consistently perform better when tested on old scales than when tested on contemporaneous scales. This may seem like 'magic' or an odd phenomenon; however, there are explanations for why this may happen. Society is consistently giving children a better and healthier environment in which to live; for example, through the advances in immunization programs and nutrition, nursery education and other factors. Thus, children are scoring better as time goes on.

The room/environment in which a child is assessed is also fundamentally important: children must not be distracted by their parents; there must be a child-friendly environment, where for example the table is set at an appropriate level for the age of the child; the child must not be distracted by any extraneous stimuli, so that they will apply natural curiosity to the particular part of the assessment they are being given; the child must use the same maternal tongue as the language of the assessment. Even cultural differences within a language can be important for some measures. For example, 'how long does it take you to go one block?' would mean something to a child from North America but be meaningless to a child from Europe.

When making assessments, ideally the same observers should be used for all children in a particular cohort/study. Of course this would be impracticable and inappropriate across international studies and, although I have personally assessed more than 600 children in this research field, and found it enjoyable, such assessments are potentially fatiguing to the observer – especially with very young children who can be quite wearing/challenging in their efforts to move on from what they are supposed to be doing.

Other problems that arise include the all-important failure of appropriate matching criteria between the index ART child and the control/compared-to child. The most important aspects to affect neurodevelopmental outcome included birth weight, sex and maturity, followed by maternal educational level and parental socioeconomic status. Then there are further factors that are potentially important, such as whether or not the child attended nursery or school. A child should not be assessed if they have a concurrent illness. If the child has a specific disability such as deafness, inevitably the effect on the child's development will not solely extend to the linguistics scale, as learning by hearing is the commonest way in which children who are in education acquire knowledge. Another flaw in some studies is to mix singleton children with those from higher-order births.

Furthermore, there are problems with the matching of cases and controls, which could include what is referred to as response bias. A simple example would be when families were contacted, if in the index case group a significant percentage attended (such as ideally 90% or more of families) whereas in the control group only 50% attended. Unless it is possible to analyze information about those who did not attend in order to compare the demographics of both groups, one cannot be confident that there is no bias in the families that attend which may be contributing to relative positive distortion in favor of the ART child, or a negative distortion since those families that are more likely to attend may have children who they are particularly concerned about.

There is another concept which needs to be considered in neurodevelopmental outcome studies. For each month of age the child gains they become potentially more skilled. Thus the limitations of human ability in children of younger age entails potentially less validity of neurodevelopmental assessment as a predictor of adult ability. For example, the typical predictability in terms of correlation coefficient of an assessment of a child of 1 year old has an r value of 0.30 whereas it has been shown that the neurodevelopmental abilities of 5-year-olds are much stronger predictors of adult ability. This is not to say that assessment of younger children is invalid; it is merely less useful for prediction of ultimate neurodevelopment. Nonetheless, by the age of 3 one can reliably assess a range of aspects of children's development. For instance, an average 3-year-old will have a vocabulary of approximately 300 words and will be able to communicate about their needs and wishes, often combining words into simple phrases and sentences. A child of this age will also be able to manipulate simple shapes, copy simple two-dimensional figures and engage in symbolic play using a variety of materials. Several formal measures of verbal processing and visual spatial cognitive ability can be made from 2 years 6 months upwards, which allow for comparison within developmental age bands and across ages or over time with the same tool.

What are the key determinants of neurodevelopmental outcome? From the known literature the developmental prognosis of the child is directly linked to: birth weight; maturity at birth (for each extra day and week of pregnancy the developmental prognosis is superior); parental – and especially maternal – educational level of attainment (regardless of whether she is working or not); then there are lists of other factors which potentially contribute with diminishing significance.

On the basis of the known literature it is fair to say that if the child is born after assisted conception and is a 'mature' child, i.e. born 34 weeks or above in gestation (it has been known in the UK for some time that the developmental outcome for a child of over 34 weeks' gestation is the same as that of a term baby) then the assisted conception has no relevance/ negative effect on the child's development. The burden of problems in ART conception is if the child is born prematurely as a result of being born from a higher-order birth or because of being born prematurely, owing to maternal or fetal reasons. It is also true to say that even singleton ART-conceived children are slightly lighter for dates than their naturally conceived peers, so as a population there would be a skewing effect on neurodevelopmental outcome due to this slightly reduced birth weight. Nonetheless, this is largely compensated for by such factors as those discussed above (such as the higher socioeconomic status of the ART-born children). Regarding the suggestions that there are defects due to assisted conception *per se* from the technique (of which there are a number described briefly in this book), my personal view is that the technique has no effect on the neurodevelopmental outcome.

A formal review now follows. Please note that this is not a comprehensive review; some studies are omitted because of either small size or various other design flaws. Of the English language papers reviewed, none are referred to in which there were no controls used, as they can be considered essentially uninformative. Reference has not been made to studies of children born after an oocyte or sperm donation where the data are weak, their confounders are large and in essence the offspring's neurodevelopmental *risk* can be considered as no different from those from any other form of ART conception. The review is largely based on a (as yet unpublished) review performed by Annika and Michael Ludwig (on which Alastair Sutcliffe is co-author), which had the following strategy: essentially 736 references were reviewed, which may have seemed relevant because of words like health, intracytoplasmic sperm injection (ICSI), *in vitro* fertilization (IVF), growth and neurodevelopment, and papers were excluded if the children were less than 6 months of age but more importantly if plurality of gestation was ignored. Only 33 studies met the matching criteria. Mixing twins, triplets and singletons in a paper concerning neurodevelopment is not wise unless there is an appropriately sized group appropriately matched in each of the study in both study arms. This is commonly not found in existing publications. Thus it can be seen that this review is quite concise; however, it does give important and positive messages and these can be stated fairly authoritatively on the basis of the known literature (which is adequate for the conclusions of this chapter).

Some of the papers that are reviewed here describe predominantly neurological findings (Table 5.1)[1–10] and others describe predominantly neurodevelopmental findings (Table 5.2)[1,3,4,6,7,9-19]. Herein are specific comments on some of the papers reflecting their relative strengths and weaknesses.

Kerryn Saunders and colleagues in Australia conducted a fairly detailed review of IVF children born in the State of Victoria between January 1989 and July 1991 and these were compared with naturally conceived children[8]. The study did not demonstrate an independent effect of IVF on the growth and physical outcome of the children and, although two children were described who had cerebral palsy, these were twins and therefore will not be discussed further. This was one of the early studies and involved 196 singleton IVF children and 113 control children who were singleton.

Prior to this Joseph Brandes and colleagues in Israel had studied 116 IVF children born between February 1985 and March 1989 with 116 non-IVF control children[18]. These were matched and the developmental indices of the IVF infants were within the normal range, and did not differ from those of their matched controls.

Koivurova et al. in Finland studied a cohort of 299 IVF children born between 1990 and 1995 and compared these children with a cohort of 558 controls representing the general population randomly chosen from the Finnish medical birth register and matched appropriately for sex, year of birth, area of residence, parity, maternal age and social class[11]. Of these, 150 were singleton IVF children and these were compared with 558 singleton control children. No statistically significant differences were found in the psychomotor development between cohorts. However, infant mortality in the IVF group was twice the national rate and the infants were also at a higher risk of being small in terms of weight and height. Therefore, Koivurova et al. concluded that the growth of IVF children was behind that of control children, but psychomotor development was normal. They thought that postnatal health was poorer because of problems in the neonatal period.

In a birth registry study performed in Denmark, Lidegaard and colleagues looked at the Danish national IVF registry derived from the national registry of patients and the central register of psychiatric diseases which included all discharge diagnoses from physical and psychiatric hospitals and clinics, respectively. There was a 7-year study period[1]. This study involved 442 349 singleton non-IVF and 6052 IVF children. In the IVF group there was a significantly increased risk of cerebral palsy with a rate ratio of 1.8 and of sleeping disturbances with a rate ratio of 2.0.

Table 5.1 Neurological health of children born after assisted reproduction (organized in reverse chronological order of report publication)

Author	Age	Neurological health
Lidegaard et al., 2005[1]	IVF: 4.5 years NC: 4.1 years (followed up at these mean ages)	Cerebral palsy: IVF: 20 cases → 3.3/1000, SC: 819 cases → 1.9/1000, RR: 1.8 (95% CI 1.2–2.8)
Pinborg et al., 2004[2]	2–7 years IVF or ICSI twins: mean 4.2 ± 1.7 NC twins: 4.4 ± 1.7 (p < 0.001) IVF or ICSI singletons: 4.1 ± 1.7 (NS)	Crude prevalence of children with neurological sequelae: IVF twins: 8.8/1000, SC twins: 9.6/1000, IVF singletons 8.2/1000 No differences in OR of neurological sequelae, cerebral palsy, mental retardation with and without adjustment for child's sex and year of birth, no difference between IVF vs. ICSI twins and IVF vs. ICSI singletons Independent risk factors for neurological sequelae in all three cohorts and for twins alone: low birth weight or prematurity (OR all: 2.3 (95% CI 1.6–3.2), OR twins: 1.9 (95% CI 1.4–2.8)), male sex (OR all: 2.0 (95% CI 1.4–2.8), OR twins: 1.9 (95% CI 1.3–2.8)) After adjustment for low birth weight or prematurity: IVF or maternal age > 35 or being a twin: no influence
Ponjaert-Kristoffersen et al., 2004[3]	ICSI: 5.2 years NC: 5.4 years	No differences after detailed neurological examination

continued

93

Table 5.1 Continued

Author	Age	Neurological health
Pinborg et al., 2003[4]	3–4 years	No differences regarding severe neurological disabilities (mental retardation, cerebral palsy, infantile autism, Asperger's syndrome): IVF twins: 0.88%, IVF singletons: 1.11%, NC twins: 1.25%
Ericson et al., 2002[5]	1–11 years	OR for being hospitalized for specific diagnosis, IVF children versus NC, stratified for year of birth, maternal age, parity and smoking: Cerebral palsy: OR 1.69 (95% CI 1.06–2.68) Epilepsy: OR 1.54 (95% CI 1.10–2.15) Mental retardation, developmental disturbances: OR not significantly increased
Stromberg et al., 2002[6]	18 months to 14 years	The overall risk of disability was increased in children born after IVF, even after exclusion of twins. IVF 2%, NC 1%, OR (all IVF): 1.8 (95% CI 1.3–2.2), OR (IVF singletons): 1.4 (95% CI 1.0–2.1) Cerebral palsy: all IVF children: OR 3.7 (95% CI 2.0–6.6), IVF singletons: OR 2.8 (95% CI 1.3–5.8), OR not increased for IVF twins, after stratification for gestational age and birth weight, OR 2.5 (95% CI 1.1–5.2)

continued

Table 5.1 *Continued*

Author	Age	Neurological health
		Risk factors for cerebral palsy: all cases and singletons: IVF (only for all cases significant, for singletons not significant), male sex, low birth weight, low gestational age (not maternal age)
		Risk for contact with childhood disability service: all cases and singletons: low birth weight, low gestational age, male sex (only for all cases significant, for singletons not significant)
Wennerholm *et al.*, 1998[7]	≤18 months	No differences regarding neurological disorders (Cryo 1.2%, IVF, SC: 0, NS), developmental delay (Cryo 0.8%, IVF: 0.4%, NC: 1.6%, NS) or eye disorder (Cryo 0.8%, IVF: 1.2%, SC: 0.4%, NS)
Saunders *et al.*, 1996[8]	IVF: 2.03 years NC: 2.04 years	2 IVF children with spastic diplegia; IVF status was not a significant independent risk factor
Ron-El *et al.*, 1994[9]	IVF: 36.6 months NC: 38.6 months	All children with normal neurological finding
Morin *et al.*, 1989[10]	12–30 months	No differences regarding major neurological abnormalities

IVF, *in vitro* fertilization; ICSI, intracytoplasmic sperm injection; Cryo, cryopreservation; NC, natural conception; RR, relative risk; OR, odd ratio; CI, confidence interval; NS, not significant

Table 5.2 Neurodevelopment of children born after assisted reproduction (organized in reverse chronological order of report publication)

Author	Age	Mental health and development
Lidegaard et al., 2005[1]	IVF: 4.5 years SC: 4.1 years	Sleeping disturbances increased in IVF children (RR: 2.0 (95% CI 1.2–3.3)) Other diagnosis not significantly different
Ponjaert-Kristoffersen et al., 2004[3]	ICSI: 5.2 years SC: 5.4 years	No differences in VIQ, PIQ, FSIQ VIQ, PIQ and FSIQ were not influenced by gestational age or birth weight More ICSI children scored 1SD below the mean in 3 subtests of the PIQ: object assembly, block design, mazes ($p < 0.05$), more SC children scored 1SD below the mean in subset of the VIQ: however, this is not explained and unlikely to be of relevance Motor development: ICSI lower scores than SC in GMQ and FMQ ($p < 0.05$) however, differences in different countries
Koivurova et al., 2003[11]	Monthly until 12 months; then 18 months, 2 and 3 years	No differences in psychomotor development assessed as part of the Finnish national child surveillance program
Pinborg et al., 2003[4]	3–4 years	No differences regarding speech impairment

continued

Table 5.2 *Continued*

Author	Age	Mental health and development
Place and Englert, 2003[12]	0–2 years	No differences in walking age and mean talking age
	3–5 years	Eating and sleeping disorders in all 3 groups: none
		No differences in development at 9 + 18 months, no differences between genders
		At age 3 and 5: IVF and ICSI mean IQ as well as subscale quotients significantly lower compared to SC, after adjustment for education of parents, no difference
		Shift in distribution of IQ
		Age 3: mildly delayed performance: ICSI: 19.4%, IVF: 36.7%, SC: 7.6%
		Age 3: significantly delayed performance: ICSI: 3.2%
		At age 5: mildly delayed: ICSI: 6.6% (but explained by prematurity and lower birth weight)
Stromberg et al., 2002[6]	1–14 years	Suspected developmental delay: all children: OR 4.0 (1.9–8.3), IVF singletons: 2.0 (95% CI 0.7–5.4), IVF twins:1.3 (95% CI 0.6–3.0) but this was a relatively imprecise proxy for DD, i.e. attended developmental centers or not
		Risk factors for suspected developmental delay: low birth weight (only for all cases significant, for singletons not significant), low gestational age
Sutcliffe et al., 2003[13]	UK: 17 months Australia:13 months	No differences between groups and between cohorts from UK and Australia
		No influence of sperm parameter on Griffiths score

continued

continued

Table 5.2 *Continued*

Author	Age	Mental health and development
Sutcliffe *et al.*, 2001[14]	ICSI: 17.2 months SC: 18.0 months	No differences in Griffiths score No influence of sperm parameter on Griffiths score
Sutcliffe *et al.*, 1999[15]	ICSI: 17.3 months SC: 17.6 months	No difference in Griffiths score ICSI children had a lower score for eye–hand coordination ($p < 0.05$)
Bowen *et al.*, 1998[16]	ICSI: 13.1 months IVF: 13.2 months	Bayley score: MDI significantly lower in ICSI children than in SC and IVF children ($p < 0.0001$), MDI also significantly lower in ICSI children when analyzing singletons and twins separately ($p = 0.002$, $p = 0.03$) between-group difference strong for boys ($p = 0.002$), only trend for girls ($p = 0.057$) 15% of ICSI children mildly delayed (MDI 1–2 SD below mean) [IVF: 2%, SC: 1%, $p < 0.0001$], 1% of ICSI children significantly delayed (MDI > 2 SD below mean) (none of IVF and SC) PDI no differences, but all groups lower than Bayley's standardization sample; however, data later at aged 5; healthy, with no developmental delay
Gibson *et al.*, 1998[17]	IVF: 13.2 months SC: 13.3 months	Bayley: no differences in MDI or PDI Receptive language: IVF significantly lower score than SC ($p = 0.006$) No differences in expressive language and socialization score

Table 5.2 *Continued*

Author	Age	Mental health and development
Wennerholm et al., 1998[7]	≤18 months	No difference in psychomotor development, delayed psychomotor development at 18 months: Cryo: 2.4%, IVF: 1.2%, SC: 2.0%
Ron-El et al., 1994[9]	≥28 months	No differences in General Cognitive Index – a little-known measure – very small numbers studied
Brandes et al., 1992[18]	12–45 months IVF: 22.4 months SC: 24.0 months	No differences in MDI or Stanford–Binet scales between groups Difference in MDI between singletons and multiples ($p = 0.002$) Positive correlation between the developmental indices of study and control cases and gestational age, birth weight, centiles of weight at birth and at examination, centiles of head circumference at birth and at examination, mother's education ($p = 0.003$) Negative correlation between developmental indices and the number of fetuses in each pregnancy ($p = 0.003$)
Gershoni-Baruch et al., 1991[19]	Index case: 13 months Control: 20 months	No difference in MDI between groups for singletons and twins

continued

Table 5.2 *Continued*

Author	Age	Mental health and development
Morin *et al.*, 1989[10]	12–30 months	No differences in MDI, PDI in IVF children significantly higher than in SC (*p* = 0.04) Behavior subscales of Bayley's with differences: IVF children vocalized more frequently (*p* = 0.02) and had higher levels of energy (*p* = 0.03)

IVF, *in vitro* fertilization; ICSI, intracytoplasmic sperm injection; SC, spontaneous conception; WPPS-r, Wechsler Preschool and Primary Scale–revised; VIQ, verbal intelligence quotient; PIQ, performance intelligence quotient; FSIQ, full-scale intelligence quotient; PDMS, Peabody Developmental Motor Scales; GMQ, gross motor quotient; FMQ, fine motor quotient; CBCL, child behavior checklist; Bayley, Bayley Scale of Infant Development; MDI, Mental Development Index; PDI, Psychomotor Development Index; Griffiths Scales, Griffiths Mental Development Scales

However, the incidence of mental diseases and developmental distur-bances was equal between the two groups. The reader needs to interpret these data with caution; whilst being impressive in terms of the very large numbers of cases and controls involved, one cannot rely upon the quality of the 'discharge data entry system' in Denmark and it would not detect children who had not been in hospital. Therefore, this paper will give only a partial message as to whether or not there is a problem.

In a seemingly separate study by Pinborg et al., also coming from Den-mark, questionnaires had been sent to a national cohort study of births occurring in 1997[4]. This involved 634 IVF and ICSI singletons and some-what curiously these were compared with twins. Questionnaire surveys inevitably have their weaknesses because they rely on (often non-skilled) lay people to elicit accurate medically diagnostic information. Notwith-standing this, the study did have the merits of involving a large number of children and, although predominantly orientated towards twins, neurolog-ical disability was noted in seven of the IVF/ICSI singletons. Attempts to grade their speech development and motor function would be particular-ly prone to inaccuracy because (quote) 'the mothers were asked to rate their speech development and their ability of walking/running on a five-point scale from much better, to much worse compared with children at the same age level'. Somewhat unsurprisingly, the IVF/ICSI twin mothers were more likely to assess their children's speech development better than other children at the same age. This is unsurprising because other research has demonstrated that children born to mothers who have conceived with IVF and ICSI are perceived as more positive in terms of parental satisfac-tion[20] and this would inevitably result in bias. In fact, this aspect of the study's assessment is virtually valueless. It is only reported in order to draw attention to the kind of measurement manifesting as 'science', which sometimes appears in quite respectable medical journals. Other aspects of the paper were more constructive. For example, it is not possible to 'fake' cerebral palsy; however, there would have to be much larger numbers to give a more reliable estimate of cerebral palsy rates.

Ulla-Britt Wennerholm and colleagues in Sweden conducted a study looking specifically at the health of children born after IVF with embryo cryopreservation[7]. They investigated the postnatal growth and health up to 18 months of age of these children compared with those born after stan-dard IVF with fresh embryos and those from spontaneous pregnancies. The main endpoint was growth; however, development was also one of the parameters assessed. There was no evidence of a difference between the three groups in terms of psychomotor development. This corroborates ear-lier work by Sutcliffe[21] which is open to the criticism that there was no allowance for plurality in the matching criteria. In his study the children were individually assessed with an appropriate developmental tool, which is a more costly but a more thorough way of assessing children. It was found that there was little difference between children born after embryo cryopreservation and naturally conceived children.

Frances Gibson and colleagues in Sydney conducted a study of development, behavior and temperaments of children who were conceived after IVF[17]. The development of 65 singleton infants was compared with 63 matched controls and these were compared 1 year postpartum. The Bayley behavior rating scales were used and there was a tendency for the receptive language development to be lower in the IVF infants than in the control infants. This study had the benefit of being prospective but had the disadvantage of being relatively underpowered. Another advantage of this study was the personal assessment of the children. Furthermore, the participation rate was very high, at 93% for the IVF group and 98% for the control group.

In another study from Sydney, Jennifer Bowen and colleagues studied a cohort of children who had been conceived by what was then a new form of IVF called ICSI. They compared 84 children conceived by standard IVF with 89 children conceived by ICSI and 80 children conceived naturally[16]. The Bayley scales of infant development were used. These studies suggested an inferior level of developmental achievement among ICSI children. However, the same cohort was studied at 5 years of age and found to be developmentally normal, and thus this early worry was overcome by more detailed study. The reader's attention is drawn to the comments above about the sensitivity and specificity of developmental measurement at a younger age.

Sutcliffe and colleagues, in two papers, described a national study in the UK of children born after ICSI. At a mean age of 18 months their findings were reassuring and involved 221 ICSI-conceived children and 208 naturally conceived children[14,15]. The children were assessed using Griffiths scales of mental development and no difference was found between the two groups. The advantage of this study was that it was carried out by a single observer; the disadvantage was that he was not blinded to conception status. There was a 90% participation rate in the ICSI group and nearly 100% in the control group, which were good aspects of the study design.

Considering poor-quality papers; the reader is referred to the study by Ron-El and others from Israel, which examined the development of children born after ovarian superovulation induced by long-acting gonadotropin releasing hormone (GnRH) agonists and menotropins and by IVF[9]. They used a little-heard-of developmental measure called the 'general cognitive index' to compare 26 children with 29 in the control group and found similarities in abilities between the groups. This study was underpowered but still concluded that the long-acting GnRH agonist had no clinically identifiable effect on the development of these children. This statement is hard to believe in view of the weakness of the data of that study. Whilst one would not wish to underestimate the difficulties of such studies, their validity, and their contribution to overall knowledge, is what this chapter aims to describe.

Isabel Place and Yvon Englert in Belgium described a group of 66 ICSI-conceived children compared with 52 IVF-conceived children and 59 spontaneously conceived children[12]. The formal developmental and intellectual assessment showed that, at 3 years and 5 years of age, there were striking similarities between the groups.

Another Belgian study was conducted by Ingrid Ponjaert-Kristoffersen and colleagues in collaboration with Swedish and American groups investigating the development of 5-year-old ICSI-conceived children[3]. Here they used the Weschler preschool and primary scales of intelligence and the Peabody developmental motor scale (and other tools to assess other aspects of health, which will be discussed in another chapter of this book). They studied 300 children in each group and overall there was no significant difference between the groups.

The most comprehensive assessment of neurodevelopment of 5-year-old children conceived naturally versus IVF versus ICSI was conducted by a group of which the joint scientific principle investigators were Sutcliffe and Bonduelle[22]. This study, known as the ICSI–CFO International Collaborative Study of ICSI–Child and Family outcomes, was funded by the European Union and was recently completed. It was a comprehensive assessment of the children, specific aspects of which are referred to herein. The children were assessed using the Weschler preschool and primary scales of intelligence and also the McCarthy motor scales. The group sizes were very powerful for this kind of outcome: 511 ICSI-conceived children were compared with 424 IVF-conceived children and 488 naturally conceived children. There was no evidence on the basis of these detailed assessments (which included full physical examination with audiometry screening and eye checks; Figure 5.2), which were generally conducted blinded to conception status, of any difference between the three groups due to mode of conception. This is the most comprehensive study and is reassuring, but it was not without fault. Participation rates varied (for example) and it was predetermined that children born below 32 weeks gestation would be excluded from the cohort because of the difficulty of finding valid matching criteria for these children: controls less than 32 weeks are problematic, as many exposures resulting from being looked after in neonatal units (e.g. ventilation, severe sepsis, etc.) would make it very difficult to obtain comparability between groups.

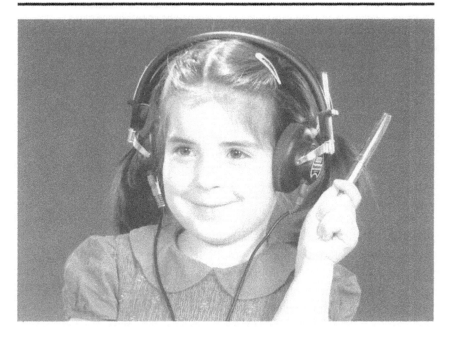

Figure 5.2 Demonstrating pure-tone audiometry screening, aged 5 years

Three large registry-based cohort studies reported an increased risk of cerebral palsy 1.7–2.8-fold in IVF children[1,5,6]. The risk of being hospitalized for epilepsy is increased significantly, 1.5-fold[5].

Stromberg and colleagues in Sweden performed a study based on a retrospective cohort looking at the neurological sequelae of children born after IVF in which they compared 5680 children born after IVF with 11 316 matched controls[6]. Data were obtained on neurological problems from the records of the Swedish developmental centers. It was found that children born after IVF were more likely to need developmental services than controls; for singletons the risk was 1.4 and the most common neurological diagnosis was cerebral palsy. Singleton children born after IVF had an increased risk of 2.8. Suspected developmental delay was increased four-fold in children born after IVF; these risks were largely due to the high frequency of twin pregnancies, low birth weight and prematurity amongst babies born after IVF.

In another large registry-based study, of 9057 IVF children, Ericson *et al.*[5] found the risk for cerebral palsy and the risk for epilepsy to be increased significantly, by 1.69 and by 1.54, respectively, in children after IVF. In a recent study Lidegaard *et al.*[1] confirmed these findings and reported the relative risk of cerebral palsy to be 1.8 in 6052 children after IVF.

Other studies that were all based on interviews or neurological examinations did not find differences regarding neurological abnormalities[3,8–10]. It has to be noted that the cohort size of these studies were much smaller and the children were only up to 5 years old.

In conclusion, there is no reliable evidence to suggest that ART has any direct bearing upon the neurodevelopmental wellbeing of children as an independent risk factor. There remains the risk of cerebral palsy as a result of prematurity and low birth weight. However, if only singleton babies were born, this risk would be further substantially reduced. Overall, this is one of the most important positive findings from the studies of ART progeny and represents good news for all who are stakeholders in ART.

As the large registry-based studies with a longer follow-up period show a strong evidence of an increase in neurological problems after ART, while those studies that show no increase are of smaller sample sizes and shorter follow-up periods, the evidence seems sufficient for an increase in neurological problems after ART (Figure 5.1). But there is no evidence for an increase in those problems in IVF twins compared to spontaneously conceived twins.

REFERENCES

1. Lidegaard O, Pinborg A, Andersen AN. Imprinting diseases and IVF: Danish National IVF cohort study. Hum Reprod 2005; 20: 950–4
2. Pinborg A, Loft A, Schmidt L, et al. Neurological sequelae in twins born after assisted conception: controlled national cohort study. Br Med J 2004; 329: 311
3. Ponjaert-Kristoffersen I, Tjus T, Nekkebroeck J, et al. Psychological follow-up study of 5-year-old ICSI children. Hum Reprod 2004; 19: 2791–7
4. Pinborg A, Loft A, Schmidt L, Andersen AN. Morbidity in a Danish national cohort of 472 IVF/ICSI twins, 1132 non-IVF/ICSI twins and 634 IVF/ICSI singletons: health-related and social implications for the children and their families. Hum Reprod 2003; 18: 1234–43
5. Ericson A, Nygren KG, Olausson PO, Kallen B. Hospital care utilization of infants born after IVF. Hum Reprod 2002; 17: 929–32
6. Stromberg B, Dahlquist G, Ericson A, et al. Neurological sequelae in children born after in-vitro fertilisation: a population-based study. Lancet 2002; 359: 461–5
7. Wennerholm UB, Albertsson-Wikland K, Bergh C, et al. Postnatal growth and health in children born after cryopreservation as embryos. Lancet 1998; 351: 1085–90
8. Saunders K, Spensley J, Munro J, Halasz G. Growth and physical outcome of children conceived by in vitro fertilization. Pediatrics 1996; 97: 688–92

9. Ron-El R, Lahat E, Golan A, et al. Development of children born after ovarian superovulation induced by long-acting gonadotropin-releasing hormone agonist and menotropins, and by in vitro fertilization. J Pediatr 1994; 125: 734–7

10. Morin NC, Wirth FH, Johnson DH, et al. Congenital malformations and psychosocial development in children conceived by in vitro fertilization. J Pediatr 1989; 115: 222–7

11. Koivurova S, Hartikainen AL, Sovio U, et al. Growth, psychomotor development and morbidity up to 3 years of age in children born after IVF. Hum Reprod 2003; 18: 2328–36

12. Place I, Englert Y. A prospective longitudinal study of the physical, psychomotor, and intellectual development of singleton children up to 5 years who were conceived by intracytoplasmic sperm injection compared with children conceived spontaneously and by in vitro fertilization. Fertil Steril 2003; 80: 1388–97

13. Sutcliffe AG, Saunders K, McLachlan R, et al. A retrospective case–control study of developmental and other outcomes in a cohort of Australian children conceived by intracytoplasmic sperm injection compared with a similar group in the United Kingdom. Fertil Steril 2003; 79: 512–16

14. Sutcliffe AG, Taylor B, Saunders K, et al. Outcome in the second year of life after in-vitro fertilisation by intracytoplasmic sperm injection: a UK case–control study. Lancet 2001; 357: 2080–4

15. Sutcliffe AG, Taylor B, Li J, et al. Children born after intracytoplasmic sperm injection: population control study. Br Med J 1999; 318: 704–5

16. Bowen JR, Gibson FL, Leslie GI, Saunders DM. Medical and developmental outcome at 1 year for children conceived by intracytoplasmic sperm injection. Lancet 1998; 351: 1529–34

17. Gibson FL, Ungerer JA, Leslie GI, et al. Development, behaviour and temperament: a prospective study of infants conceived through in-vitro fertilization. Hum Reprod 1998; 13: 1727–32

18. Brandes JM, Scher A, Itzkovits J, et al. Growth and development of children conceived by in vitro fertilization. Pediatrics 1992; 90: 424–9

19. Gershoni-Baruch R, Scher A, Itskovitz J, et al. The physical and psychomotor development of children conceived by IVF and exposed to high-frequency vaginal ultrasonography (6.5 MHz) in the first trimester of pregnancy. Ultrasound Obstet Gynecol 1991; 1: 21–8

20. Barnes J, Sutcliffe AG, Kristofferson I, et al. The influence of assisted reproduction on family functioning and children's socio-emotional development: results from a European study. Hum Reprod 2004; 19: 1480–7

21. Sutcliffe AG, D'Souza SW, Cadman J, et al. Outcome in children from cryopreserved embryos. Arch Dis Child 1995; 72: 290–3

22. Bonduelle M, Wennerholm UB, Loft A, et al. A multi-centre cohort study of the physical health of 5-year-old children conceived after intracytoplasmic sperm injection, in vitro fertilization and natural conception. Hum Reprod 2005; 20: 413–19

Chapter 6

Psychosocial aspects of ART

Jacqueline Barnes

INTRODUCTION

The psychosocial implications of assisted reproductive technology (ART) can begin for families many years prior to the birth of a child. Any type of assisted reproductive therapy may be associated with long periods of parental stress, compared to natural conception, which could influence adaptation to the parental role, parental relationships, parent–child relationships and children's socioemotional development. Investigations of families created by ART have focused much of their attention on identifying potential risks to child development, mediated by parental stress, associated parental mental health problems, problematic family relationships, difficulties with parenting and distorted parental cognitions. To put it simply, it has been assumed that the significant and increasingly common stressor – infertility – and the ensuing *in vitro* fertilization (IVF) or other ART experience may disrupt early parenting styles and impact in a number of ways on family life and consequently on children's development[1]. This is evident in a recently developed measure, the Parenting After Infertility (PAI) survey[2], which is composed of four sub-scales labeled: 'emotional aspects of infertility'; 'being a perfect parent'; 'disclosure of children's origins'; and 'overprotection of children'.

A particular prevailing and reasonable expectation has been that, because children conceived using ART are born to couples after years of investment and waiting, with the ensuing stresses, the children may be seen as more vulnerable by their parents, which could lead to overprotective parenting. This in turn may have an impact on children's behavior. Other factors to consider are that ART parents are on average older than other parents and many of the pregnancy outcomes are multiple births, known to place children at risk for not only developmental problems but also behavioral difficulties. This chapter discusses the stresses that parents who have experienced ART in its many forms might encounter, both prior to their child's birth and subsequently, and the research evidence related to these stresses as they impact on parenting behavior, parent–child relationships and children's socioemotional development.

SPECIFIC SOURCES OF FAMILY STRESS

Infertility

Infertility followed by parenthood will be both an immense relief and a jolt of reality, as the daily parenting tasks replace years of longing for a child in a rather abstract way. The first and possibly most important stress to consider is that related to the long period of infertility that usually precedes ART[3]. Infertility can have a detrimental effect on women's self-identity[4], and many report that infertility is the worst experience of their life[5]. A review of the international literature found that consequences identified for women include: anxiety, depression, lowered life satisfaction, frustration, grief, fear, guilt, helplessness, reduced job performance, marital duress, dissolution of relationships and abandonment, economic hardship, loss of social status, social stigma, social isolation and alienation, community ostracism and physical violence[6].

However, it may be equally or even more stressful for men, although studies have generally found that they report less stress than women[7,8]. In the past 10 years there has been increasing use of intracytoplasmic sperm injection (ICSI)[9,10], primarily for the treatment, at least in the past, of male-factor infertility. Many men find a diagnosis of infertility to be an unexpected shock. Nobody wants such a diagnosis but it seems to be particularly difficult for men in relation to their sense of self. In all of the recent discussions about infertility there is still an assumption that its causes are most likely to be found within women so that when men are told that there is a sperm problem, typically they are quite unprepared[11]. While there are other reactions to male infertility, for most men it comes 'out of the blue' and they may not have ways of dealing with what they are being told – ways that are available to some women. Male socialization against experiencing and expressing weakness means that men often cannot find the words to talk about losses. In addition, men who do feel upset about infertility are living lives in which they keep their upset feelings a secret[12]. In addition, men may be secretive about male infertility because they feel that others will link their infertility with impotence and lack of masculinity.

Thus there is a possibility that male factor 'problems' may lead to more secrecy about disclosure and potentially more marital discord[13].

Parents at particular risk may be those who have not worked through their conflict towards infertility by the time they become parents, in which case the child may act as a 'narcissistic injury'[3]*, constantly reminding at least one parent of her or his infertility and potentially creating an asymmetry between the parents which could result in marital discord and disagreements about child-rearing.

ART procedures

While the experience of ART could be expected to relieve some of the emotional concerns associated with infertility, ART treatments are themselves also likely to raise levels of anxiety, with clinical depression possible if treatment fails[7,8]. It would not be surprising if these emotional reactions lead to parenting problems once the baby arrives. Research over the past two decades has shown psychosocial distress among random samples of infertile couples undergoing infertility treatment[14], indicating that the experience may result in depressive and anxiety symptoms[15] and other psychosocial problems[16-18]. Reflecting the concerns that men may have about infertility, while the women in a retrospective study conducted in Germany of 281 couples reported more treatment-related stress than men, when the family had undergone ICSI men described more subjective responsibility for the impact of childlessness on family life[19]. In view of the risk for this kind of mental health problem, and subsequent anxiety once pregnancy is achieved, it has been suggested that there may be parenting problems[20], either because the depression persists even on attaining parenthood or because the new child may subconsciously be 'blamed' for the experience of being so low.

A recent Swedish study comparing couples who achieved pregnancy either through natural means or using IVF found differences in the emotions of both the mothers and the fathers[21,22]. They concluded that negative feelings related to infertility are not easily overcome even though an IVF treatment is successful and parenthood achieved. Interviews were

---

*'Narcissistic injury' describes damage to the individuals' experience of their 'real self'. In its more extreme forms, individuals are left with no awareness at all of who they really are. In the less extreme variations of this disorder, there is often a vague comprehension of the real self but also a rejection of it. A mother who has not had her narcissistic needs met may unconsciously use the infant to satisfy her own needs. She loves the child as an extension of herself, rather than for his/herself. For more details see Miller A. The Drama of Being a Child. London: Virago, 1981

conducted with 57 women pregnant after IVF, 55 male partners and 43 women who had conceived naturally with 39 male partners. They completed a number of scales measuring personality traits, anxiety, emotional responses to pregnancy, marital adjustment and recall of reactions to infertility when pregnancy was on average 13 weeks (range 11–17 weeks). The IVF women had more muscular tension and irritability than the control women during pregnancy. Anxiety about losing the pregnancy was stronger among both the IVF women and the men from early to late pregnancy compared to the controls. In addition, associations were found between a high degree of previous infertility distress and high levels of pregnancy-related anxiety among the IVF parents to be, both male and female. The IVF men had more somatic anxiety, indirect aggression, feelings of guilt and more detachment, and they tended to have more psychic anxiety than the control men. However, there were also indications of less stress, in that the IVF women were less concerned about the child's gender than the control women, and they were also less worried about possible 'loss of freedom' in their future lives as parents. The IVF men were more anxious that the baby might be injured during birth compared to the control men.

Becoming a parent

Since the inception of IVF, concerns about the subsequent adjustment to parenthood for the couples involved have been expressed. This has been due to the carryover of negative psychological sequelae from the experience of infertility and the process of IVF treatment[23,24], the obstetric risk of IVF[25] and the high expectations IVF parents have of themselves[26] and their child[27,28].

Having endured long periods of waiting and uncertainty about the survival of their child, parents may either hesitate to bond with their baby[29] or become insecurely attached, with the associated risks of overprotection[24] and disregard for the child's need to develop autonomy. Burns[30] proposed that, after problems in conceiving, parents are likely to be overprotective and emotionally overinvolved with their child, a style of parenting that has been associated with an increased risk of a range of disorders in children[31]. Reviewing issues related to the development of IVF children, Van Balen[25] concurred with the suggestion that one of the main concerns for families who become parents after a long, arduous and stressful period of longing is that the child might be seen as very 'precious' and subject to overprotection, going on to propose that parents may have exaggerated expectations of their child, known to be associated in non-ART families with a risk for child abuse[32]. Van Balen also proposed that, after a long period of infertility and childlessness, parents may have difficulty adapting to the reality of child-rearing. Finally, it is suggested that children conceived using IVF or other ART methods may be perceived as different by other people in the family's social network, which could also lead to overprotection and an overindulgent approach to discipline in the face of difficult behavior[20,33].

Donor and surrogacy issues

Some infertile couples are able to conceive through donor sperm or egg, raising additional issues in relation to parenting. Golombok *et al.*[34] raised concerns about the parent–child relationship in families with children born by donor insemination, associated with the fact that the child would be unrelated genetically to one or both of his or her parents. The Warnock report[35,36] suggested that fathers could feel inadequate or excluded following the use of donor sperm, and Snowden and Snowden[37] hypothesized that using donor sperm for conception could produce 'confusion about paternity'. It is possible that this kind of ambivalence could adversely influence subsequent father–child relationships. There may be additional psychosocial stress within the family if the lack of genetic relationship with either parent is kept secret from their child[38].

Disclosure of birth details: an ongoing issue for families

Whether or not both parents are biological, all families who have conceived using ART will probably have considered whether or not to tell their child about the conception process. There appears to be a likelihood of maintaining secrecy about ART in that the majority of parents with children aged 10 years or under who had conceived using IVF had not revealed the method of conception[13,39–43]. The maintenance of family secrets is well known to present a risk in general to family functioning[44]. Secrecy has been shown to create boundaries between those who do and do not know. Holders of family secrets may experience anxiety about the possibility of disclosure and find discussion of related topics uncomfortable. In addition, there may be implications of non-disclosure for the children's socioemotional development, based on evidence from children who were adopted, given that most family secrets are revealed at some time, even if inadvertently.

It is clear that many people in the family circle are likely to know about the ART experience. For instance, one study in the USA[42] found that 98% of the parents had told somebody about their IVF experience, although 25% remained uncertain whether at any time they would tell their child. If secrets are subsequently disclosed, the previously unaware party may feel that their trust has been violated[40]. Studies of adults adopted as children have shown that it is important that they are told of their adoption at an early age and that provision of information about their genetic background helped in the development of a stable identity[45]. It has been reported that some cultures, for example in Eastern Europe, are more secretive about disclosing conception information and more uncertain about whether to inform their child, so there may be differences in the extent to which disclosure represents a family stress[46].

However, the majority of parents who have conceived through ART do intend to tell their child at some point[41,42,47]. The study by Peters et al.[47] of children conceived with either IVF or ICSI suggests that increasing openness may be becoming the norm. This UK study found that the majority of parents of 5- or 6-year-olds who responded ($n = 181$, 51% of those surveyed) had already disclosed, or wished in the future to disclose, details about the conception method to their child. The same proportion of mothers and fathers planned to inform their child in the future, but fathers on average would tell their children slightly later, at about 10 years rather than 8 or 9 years for mothers, confirming the suggestion that ART may be more problematic for fathers than mothers. The children who had already been informed by the age of 5 about their conception status were more likely to have been told by their mothers. There also seem to be factors related to the type of ART and to the presence of existing children. Children were more likely to be told if conception was by ICSI, rather than by conventional IVF, and if an only child. Parental decisions about whether or not to inform their child may be influenced by their decision to reveal the method of conception to others. Parents in this study who did not mind who knew the child's conception status (56% mothers and 53% fathers) were more likely to have already informed their child by the age of 5–6 years or intended to inform them before they became teenagers.

Multiple births and other risks to the child

If 25% of all pregnancies after IVF/ICSI are twin pregnancies, then 40% of all babies born after ART are born as part of a twin pair. Many physicians and patient couples underestimate the negative consequences of twin pregnancies.

There may be medical complications which then have an impact on the experience of parenting. Even before the birth, families who are fully informed will know that perinatal as well as maternal mortality and morbidity are increased in multiple pregnancies as compared with singleton pregnancies, owing to a higher rate of prematurity and low birth weights in the children, and to pregnancy complications in the mothers.

Furthermore, parents of multiple births have more stress, and siblings of multiples are more likely to have behavior problems[48,49].

The potential for chemical and mechanical damage is greater using ICSI than IVF, with an increased likelihood of introducing foreign material into the oocyte. Some uncontrolled outcome studies have found a higher rate of sex chromosome abnormalities[50] or delayed development[51]. Thus, when families are informed of the potential risks, they may be more anxious over time not only about the birth experience but about their children's long-term health and development, which could have an impact both on parenting behavior and on children's socioemotional development as they become aware of parental anxiety.

WHAT IS KNOWN ABOUT PARENTING AFTER ART

Parenting and family problems

It has been suggested that there may be a risk of having problematic parent-child relationships, particularly if the parents have not come to terms with their infertility[34]. Many studies that have focused on the IVF parent–child relationship[52,53] (see reference 54 for a review) have not been conclusive and Van Balen[25], after reviewing the available literature, concluded that no negative differences could be found in parent–child relationships or children's psychological development. There are, however, concerns about generalizing from some of the earlier studies that were based on small samples, and in many cases comparisons with control groups have been confined to singleton ART births; thus less is known about parenting of multiple ART families.

In the USA, 184 couples who had conceived at a clinic in Connecticut using IVF between 1982 and 1992 were sent anonymous postal questionnaires[42]. The response rate was low (31%), one indication that many families who have used IVF may wish to move on and consider themselves no different from other families. The study found that more than half the mothers (52%) but only 19% of fathers who replied experienced 'special feelings' of attachment to their IVF children which caused some difficulties regarding separation. Other investigators have found that donor insemination IVF mothers have feelings of social isolation and over-protectiveness in the early stages of their child's life[55].

In an Australian study, IVF mothers had a lower sense of self-efficacy in care-giving at 4 months postpartum, and they also reported less autonomy-promoting behavior compared with other mothers of a similar background[26]. Subsequently, this study comparing 65 children conceived using

IVF with 61 naturally conceived controls did not identify any differences between IVF and comparison families in observed parent–child attachment, nor were any differences identified in maternal sensitivity, structuring or hostility during videotaped free play[52]. However the IVF fathers expressed lower self-esteem and less marital satisfaction than those in the natural conception control group[56] although measurement of general adjustment and parenting showed no differences. At 1 year postpartum, the mothers reported an increased concern about risks to their child, and viewed their child as more special than did the control mothers[56].

A small study in the UK of parents who had conceived using IVF/gamete intra-Fallopian transfer (GIFT)[57] found that when their infants were between 1 and 2 years of age the parents reported positive feelings about their children, higher than general population norms, and were also somewhat more overprotective than the general population. Hahn and DiPietro[1] found in Taiwan that, when their children were between 3 and 7 years, IVF mothers reported a greater level of overprotectiveness than their control counterparts. While, as with all studies of child rearing following IVF treatment, it is difficult to know whether maternal protectiveness is a function of the IVF treatment specifically or of infertility in general, it does seem that there is ongoing evidence of more protection following ART. The issue of course is whether this constitutes overprotection or merely attentive, sensitive parenting.

Most of the research described has used questionnaires and it has been suggested that studies finding ART to be related to problem-free parenting may be an indication of the tendency to give socially desirable responses[24]. Some detailed observational work in a small-scale study from Belgium found that, at 2 to 3 years, those mothers who were employed and who had used IVF were less able to allow children autonomy in a problem-solving task than unemployed mothers in the IVF group, or the comparison group[24].

The European Study of Assisted Reproduction Families, including children from the UK, The Netherlands, Italy and Spain[58] compared children conceived using either donor insemination (DI, $n = 111$) or IVF ($n = 116$) with naturally conceived controls ($n = 120$) and adopted children ($n = 115$), aged between 4 and 8 years. During in-depth interviews mothers in both assisted reproduction groups and the adoptive mothers expressed lower levels of anxiety and stress than parents who had conceived naturally. The fathers in the IVF and DI groups were more involved than mothers in the naturally conceived control group. Assisted reproduction fathers were said by mothers to interact more with their child and to contribute more to parenting, especially in The Netherlands[58]. Interestingly it has been found that, while maintaining secrecy about conception may be of particular concern in egg or sperm donor families, greater wellbeing and less stress has been reported in families who used donor egg or sperm[59]. Similarly the DI parents did not differ from the control group. However, it has been noted that none of the DI parents in any of the four countries had told their child at that stage that they were conceived using the sperm of an anonymous donor, although half had told a family member[60]. When the children were followed up to the beginning of adolescence, at age 12, the IVF parents were found to have positive relationships with their children characterized by a combination of affection and appropriate control[53,61] although, as with younger children, there were some signs indicating overinvolvement of the IVF parents, compared to the control group. There were no indications of family problems in the DI families, who also reported warmth and an appropriate level of discipline and control. A small proportion (8.6%) had by then told their child about their genetic origins, most who withheld the information indicating that they were trying to protect their child from distress, and to limit the likelihood of problems in the father–child relationship[62].

Another recent large-scale multisite European study compared 439 IVF- and 541 ICSI-conceived children with 542 naturally conceived controls, examining the relative levels of stress in the family, parental wellbeing, marital discord and adaptation to their parental role[63]. Questionnaires were completed by mothers and fathers. There were no conception group differences in mothers' or fathers' wellbeing on a mental health measure including depression, anxiety, somatic symptoms and social difficulties, nor were there significant conception group differences in levels of parental distress or marital discord. On a measure of parent–child relationships, the Parental Acceptance and Rejection Questionnaire[64], mothers who had conceived using ICSI reported fewer negative, rejecting feelings towards their children than mothers in the naturally conceived group and were specifically less likely to report aggressive or hostile feelings. There were no significant differences between the ART and control groups in the fathers' responses. While there were no observations of parent–child interactions this study did obtain the children's own views of their parents using the Bene Anthony Family Relations Test[65]. There were no group effects for positive or negative feelings towards mothers. There was, however, a trend for children conceived by ICSI to express more positive feelings about their fathers than children in the other two groups.

Thus, there does not appear to be strong evidence that parents who have conceived using ART experience more family discord or other difficulties once they become parents; in fact the opposite seems to be the case, as several more recent and larger studies have concluded.

Other parenting outcomes

Evidence of potentially positive effects of ART on parenting has been identified in a number of other studies. IVF parents have been found to be
highly emotionally involved with their children[1,34,57,58,66], to feel more
competent[66] and to report less parenting stress[34,58]. In Taiwan, in a small
study comparing IVF and naturally conceived children aged 3–7 years,
Hahn and DiPietro[1] found that teachers blind to conception status rated
IVF parents as having greater emotional involvement including warmth,
although they were not rated as more intrusive or more protective.

Other aspects of family life are now being studied, such as work/home
balance. A European study investigated mothers' and fathers' commitment
to their role as a parent, and their role in work[63]. Significant effects of conception type were found on mothers' commitment to work and to parenting, and fathers' commitment to parenting. Mothers with children
conceived through IVF were less committed to their work role than the
natural conception controls, and mothers who had conceived using ICSI
were more committed to their role as a parent than either natural conception controls or the IVF group. There were no significant differences
between the groups in fathers' commitment to work.

CHILD PERSONALITY AND SOCIOEMOTIONAL DEVELOPMENT

While many of the earlier studies performed into child outcomes from
ART focused primarily on physical problems such as birth defects and neurodevelopmental outcomes, there is a growing body of information about
children's socioemotional development. As with the early studies of parenting, samples in some cases have been small[3,52] and others lack adequate
controls[67]. However, the picture that is emerging is generally positive.

It appears that in the months immediately after birth parents of IVF-
conceived infants may judge them to be temperamentally more difficult
that those conceived naturally. One Australian longitudinal study of 65
primiparous mothers undergoing IVF and 62 age-matched controls found
that, at 4 months, babies conceived with IVF were observed to be more
negative in their responses to stressful situations, and their mothers rated
them as temperamentally more difficult[26]. This was especially likely for
mothers who had undergone more than one treatment cycle. At 1 year
these children were rated by their mothers as having more behavioral difficulties[68]. However, no differences between IVF and naturally conceived

children were identified by researchers during test-taking at that age, leading the authors to conclude that it was parental anxiety that led the mothers of IVF children to be more aware of minor behavioral problems. Observations of the mothers and children in the Ainsworth Strange Situation, designed to look at the security of the infants' attachment to their mother in stressful conditions, found that most of the IVF (and control) children were securely attached, with no difference between the groups[52].

Looking at slightly older children, observations during a mother–child interaction task did not identify any differences at 24–30 months between IVF- and naturally conceived children[24]. Similarly, using parental report studies no differences were found in behavioral or emotional problems between IVF and naturally conceived controls in small studies conducted in a number of different countries including Sweden[69], Belgium[24], The Netherlands[66] and Taiwan[1]. Indeed, in The Netherlands, IVF mothers rated their 2–4-year-olds as less obstinate than other mothers[66]. A large, uncontrolled postal and telephone survey was conducted in the USA of 743 school-aged children ranging in age from 4 to 14 years conceived using IVF, representing all those children born at one institute in Virginia between 1981 and 1990[67]. This study is one of the few that included multiple births (94, representing 37 twin pairs, four sets of triplets and two sets of quadruplets). Using the Achenbach Child Behavior Checklist (CBCL) completed by parents, the Teacher Report form and, for the older children, the Youth Self Report Form, they were compared to a national sample. With an overall 84% response rate it was found that the IVF children had similar levels of behavior problems to national norms and, while not significant, the IVF group had a greater percentage of both girls and boys in the normal range and fewer above the clinical cut-off than the control group for every domain of the scale. The multiple births did not differ from the singletons. A study of children aged between 6 months and 4 years born after egg donation, compared to IVF children, found no differences in the proportion with sleeping or eating problems, and the egg donation parents were in fact slightly less concerned about their children's behavior[70].

A UK study of 113 children conceived using ICSI found similarly that these mothers rated their children as having fewer behavioral problems than naturally conceived controls[71]. At the age of 2–3 years the children conceived through ICSI had a significantly lower mean Intensity Score on the Eyberg Child Behavior Inventory and a larger proportion of the control group were above the cut-off, indicating marked behavior problems. Mean total problem scores were also significantly lower among ICSI-conceived children than the normally conceived controls. Individual behaviors were examined and a quarter were significantly more likely for the control children than those conceived by ICSI. In particular, control children were rated by their mothers as more likely to exhibit a number of externalizing behaviors such as 'yell or scream', 'lie', 'provoke other children' and 'physically fight with friends'.

In Australia, Kovacs and colleagues[72] used the CBCL[73] to compare children conceived by DI to adoptees and naturally conceived children when they were between 6 and 8 years of age, finding no differences between the groups. A larger European study, including ICSI and IVF children from the UK, Belgium, Denmark and Sweden and naturally conceived controls looked at parental reports of behavior problems at 5 years[63]. There was no evidence of any differences between the three groups in total temperament, based on the McDevitt and Carey Scale[74] according to mothers or fathers, nor were there any differences on the basis of the Difficult Child scale of the Parenting Stress Index[75], total behavior problems as rated on the CBCL, or the proportion of children above the clinical cut-off point of the CBCL.

The European Study of Assisted Reproduction families, comparing children conceived through IVF, by donor insemination, adopted children and naturally conceived controls found no differences in behavior problems between these groups, based on questionnaires completed by mothers and by teachers[34,58]. This was reflected in the children's own reports of their self-esteem, which again were similar across groups. A small Belgian sample was followed up when the children were 8–9 years, with questionnaires completed by mothers, fathers and teachers[41]. The ratings of parents were no different in the IVF and control groups, nor were teacher reports different, although there was a tendency for teachers to report more problems for the IVF group. This study was interesting, however, in that behavior problems were related to whether or not the details of their conception had been disclosed to the children. One-quarter (7/27) of the parents had told their children and those children who had been told had higher mean scores on the CBCL internalizing problems scale, indicating problems such as anxiety and depression, and the total problem score compared to those who had not been informed.

Other studies investigating the issue of disclosure have focused mainly on DI families, finding that DI children aged 4–8 who knew their conception method had less frequent and less severe disputes with their mothers than those who had not been told[58]. However, the team did not find any relationship between secrecy and children's emotional or behavioral problems for IVF or DI children in the families from The Netherlands[40], suggesting that cultural factors interact with family secrecy in terms of its implications for children.

There is less information about older children and adolescents. One controlled study in Israel of children aged 9–10 years[76] found evidence of poorer school adjustment. Fifty-one children conceived using IVF were compared with 51 naturally conceived controls, matched for age, gender, birth order and socioeconomic status. Based on teachers' ratings the IVF group, and especially the boys, were judged to have poorer socioemotional adjustment. The children themselves completed a number of self-report measures, those conceived by IVF describing significantly more anxiety and depression and more aggression with peers than naturally conceived controls. However, the UK group from the European Study of Assisted Reproduction Families has been followed up to the age of 12 years and there continue to be no indications of any behavioral or emotional problems, compared to controls[53,61].

CONCLUSIONS

The results of most of the research described suggest that children conceived using ICSI or IVF, including those for whom either sperm or oocyte have been donated, are not at greater risk of developing problem behaviors, nor are their families showing signs of identifiable stress or strain. If anything, the children are less likely to be said by parents to have any difficulties, and there is less hostility in parent–child relationships than in families where conception has occurred naturally.

It is possible either that parents who have been through the process of ART are making greater efforts to manage and support children they have struggled to conceive, or are more tolerant of behavior that other parents find difficult. This is likely to be beneficial in the short term in that criticism and harsh parenting in the early years is a risk factor for the development of conduct problems later[77]. However, if parents are being too tolerant during the early years, once their children are older it may lead to difficulties, when behavior should be checked more appropriately. Only a handful of studies have included older children and some of these have not been controlled. Nothing is really known yet about the teenage years.

In the long term, issues such as commitment to being a parent in relation to being an adult in the world of work may become more important to families who initially had only one commitment, to conceive. The study of Barnes et al.[63] found that mothers who had conceived using ICSI were markedly more committed to being a parent than the control mothers or the mothers who had experienced IVF, and equally less committed to the role of worker outside the home. Duncan and Edwards[78] have identified three 'gendered moral rationalities' used by women to explain their roles, based on identities and responsibilities to children, those who see themselves as primarily a mother, those who see themselves primarily as a worker and those with an integrated mother–worker role. The mothers who had experienced ICSI were closest to the primarily mother identity. They were also less committed to their role in the workplace, compared to either the IVF group or the control group. This may indeed have some implications in years to come. Women who have negated their role in the 'outside world' in order to commit to parenting may, especially when the lack of conception was related to infertility of their partner rather than themselves, regret their dedication as they see their chances of career development receding. Thus, it is vital to follow these families as their children grow and the families have different priorities.

Overall, there is no indication that major parenting or child difficulties are a likely consequence of conception using any of the many types of ART now available to families, although the effort to be 'super parents' may cause long-term strain and influence the balance of power in the families. However, there are many provisos to this general conclusion. Much of the work is based on small groups who are in some sense self-selected, potentially those families who feel most positive about their ART experience. One cannot insist that families 'repay' medical advances by reporting on their experiences and many may wish, possibly sensibly, to move on and behave as families who have conceived by natural conception. They do not consider that they are in any way different or a suitable case for research investigation. While one can understand why they may not want to be placed under scrutiny by teams of researchers, the questions that their children may raise could in the long term be more challenging.

A long-term issue as children grow older is the question of disclosure. Studies are beginning to investigate this in relation to children's emotional wellbeing but it will become more problematic as children become adolescents to involve them in research studies if their parents have decided on complete secrecy. These are the families who will almost certainly have refused to take part in research, even if they did agree when their children were younger. In the teenage years issues of self-identity come to the fore and it is not inconceivable that a large proportion of the children born after sperm or gamete donation will eventually hear something from someone in the family. Most of the parents had told family members or close friends. Once these secrets emerge, and children react to being kept in the dark, there is potential for marked family discord and emotional difficulties such as depression or anger.

Cultural implications of ART may also need further investigation. In general a wide range of areas have been conducting research with ART families and their children, including Australia, the USA, Western Europe and the Far East. However, Cook et al.[46] found that the parent–child relationship and child adjustment following IVF may be different depending on the cultural milieu. They identified more difficulties in Eastern Europe than in Western European countries. More collaborative investigations will need to be designed to incorporate countries with different religious beliefs, with different approaches to the roles of men and women, and with different approaches to the autonomy and independence of children and youngsters. This may lead to a more complex, and potentially more interesting examination of what it means to overcome infertility with the help of modern medical advances, and what it means to be the product of such developments when one grows and develops.

Up to this point the questions asked about the psychosocial implications of ART have been somewhat mundane. Do parents experience more stress? Are they more protective of their 'precious' children? Do these possibly pampered children have more behavioral or emotional problems? We have been able to answer 'No' to these. In the future the more complex psychological aspects of parental identity and children's self-concept deserve and will surely receive more attention.

REFERENCES

1. Hahn CS, DiPietro JA. In vitro fertilization and the family: quality of parenting, family-functioning, and child psychosocial adjustment. Dev Psychol 2001; 37: 37–48
2. Frances-Fischer JE, Lightsey OR. Parenthood after primary fertility. Fam J 2003; 11: 117–28
3. Mushin DN, Spensley JC, Barreda-Hanson MC. Children of IVF. Clin Obstet Gynecol 1985; 12: 865–76
4. Miall CE. The stigma of involuntary childlessness. Soc Probl 1986; 33: 268–82
5. Van Balen F, Inhorn M. Interpreting infertility: a view from the social sciences. In: Inhorn M, Van Balen F, eds. Infertility Around the Globe: New Thinking on Childlessness, Gender, and Reproductive Technologies. London: University of California Press, 2002: 3–32
6. McDonald Evens E. A global perspective on infertility: an under recognized public health issue. Carolina Papers in International Health, No. 18. Chapel Hill, NC: University of North Carolina, 2004
7. Eugster A, Vingerhoets A. Psychological aspects of in vitro fertilization: a review. Soc Sci Med 1999; 48: 575–89
8. Golombok S. Psychological functioning in infertility patients. Hum Reprod 1992; 7: 208–12
9. Nygren KG, Nyboe Andersen A. Assisted reproductive technology in Europe, 1999. Results generated from European registers by ESHRE. Hum Reprod 2002; 17: 3260–74
10. Sutcliffe AG. Intracytoplasmic sperm injection and other aspects of new reproductive technologies. Arch Dis Child 2000; 83: 98–101

11. de Kretser DM. Emotional impact of male fertility on men. http://www.andrologyaustralia.org/infertility/emotionalimpact/initialreaction.htm. Accessed 13 July 2005

12. Zoldbrod A. Men, Women and Infertility: Intervention and Treatment Strategies. New York: Lexington Books, 1993

13. McWhinnie A. Outcome for families created by assisted conception programmes. J Assist Reprod Genet 1996; 13: 363–5

14. Wright J, Allard M, Lecours A, Sabourin S. Psychosocial distress and infertility: a review of controlled research. Int J Fertil 1989; 34: 126–42

15. Klock SC, Greenfeld DA. Psychological status of in vitro fertilization patients during pregnancy: a longitudinal study. Fertil Steril 2000; 73: 1159–64

16. Andrew FM, Abbey A, Halman LJ. Stress from infertility, marriage factors, and subjective wellbeing of wives and husbands. J Health Soc Behav 1991; 32: 238–63

17. Berg BJ, Wilson JF. Psychological functioning across stages of treatment for infertility. J Behav Med 1991; 14: 11–26

18. Daniluk JC. Infertility: Intrapersonal and interpersonal impact. Fertil Steril 1988; 57: 350–6

19. Beutel M, Kupfer J, Kirchmeyer P, et al. Treatment-related stresses and depression in couples undergoing assisted reproductive treatment by IVF or ICSI. Andrologia 1999; 31: 27–35

20. Bernstein J. Parenting after infertility. J Perinat Neonat Nurs 1990; 4: 11–23

21. Hjelmstedt A, Widstrom AM, Wramsby H, et al Personality factors and emotional responses to pregnancy among IVF couples in early pregnancy: a comparative study. Acta Obstet Gynecol Scand 2003; 82: 152–61

22. Hjelmstedt A, Widstrom AM, Wramsby H, Collins, A. Patterns of emotional responses to pregnancy, experience of pregnancy and attitudes to parenthood among IVF couples: a longitudinal study. J Psychosom Obstet Gynaecol 2003; 24: 153–62

23. Mahlstedt PP. Psychological issues of infertility and assisted reproductive technology. Urol Clin North Am 1994; 21: 557–66

24. Colpin H, Demyttenaere K, Vandemeulebroecke L. New reproductive technology and the family. The parent–child relationship following in vitro fertilization. J Child Psychol Psychiatry 1995; 36: 1429–41

25. Van Balen F. Development of IVF children. Dev Rev 1998; 18: 30–46

26. McMahon CA, Ungerer JA, Tennant C, Saunders D. Psychosocial adjustment and the quality of the mother–child relationship at four months postpartum after conception by in vitro fertilization. Fertil Steril 1997; 68: 492–500

27. Hammer-Burns L. Infertility as boundary ambiguity: one theoretical perspective. Fam Process 1987; 26: 359–72

28. Roegiers L, Delaisi de Parseval G. [Les cigognes en crise: desires d'enfant et éthique relationnelle en fecundation in vitro] Child wish and relational ethics in in vitro fertilization. Brussels: De Boeck, 1994

29. Pullan-Watkins K. Reference Books on Family Issues: Vol. 2: Parent–child Attachment: A Guide to Research. (Garland Reference Library on Social Science 388). New York: Garland, 1987

30. Burns LH. An exploratory study of perceptions of parenting after infertility. Fam Sys Med 1990; 8: 177–89

31. Thomasgard MT, Shonkoff JP, Metz WP, Edelbrock C. Parent–child relationship disorders. Part II. The vulnerable child syndrome and its relation to parental overprotection. Dev Behav Pediatr 1995; 16: 251–6

32. Milner JS. Assessing physical child abuse risk: The Child Abuse Potential Inventory. Clin Child Abuse Rev 1994; 14: 547–83

33. Sokoloff BZ. Alternative methods of reproduction. Effects on the child. Clin Pediatr 1987; 26: 11–17

34. Golombok S, Cook R, Bish A, Murray C. Families created by the new reproductive technologies; quality of parenting and emotional development of the children. Child Dev 1995; 66: 285–98

35. Warnock M. Report of the Committee of Inquiry into Human Fertilization and Embryology. London, UK: Her Majesty's Stationery Office, 1984

36. Warnock M. Ethics, decision-making and social policy. Comm Care 1987; 685: 18–23

37. Snowden E, Snowden R. Families created through donor insemination. In: Daniels K, Haimes E, eds. Donor Insemination. International Social Science Perspectives. Cambridge: Cambridge University Press, 1998; 33–52

38. Daniels K, Taylor K. Secrecy and openness in donor insemination. Politics Life Sci 1993; 12: 155–70

39. Braverman AM, Boxer AS, Corson SL, et al. Characteristics and attitudes of parents of children born with the use of assisted reproductive technology. Fertil Steril 1998; 70: 860–5

40. Brewaeys A, Golombok S, Naaktgeboren N, et al. Donor insemination: Dutch parents' opinions about confidentiality and donor anonymity and the emotional adjustment of their children. Hum Reprod 1997; 12: 1591–7

41. Colpin H, Soenen S. Parenting and psychosocial development of IVF children: a follow-up study. Hum Reprod 2002; 17: 1116–23

42. Greenfeld DA, Ort SI, Greenfeld DG, et al. Attitudes of IVF parents regarding the IVF experience and their children. J Assist Reprod Genet 1996; 13: 266–74

43. Olivennes F, Kerbrat V, Rufat P, et al. Follow-up of a cohort of 422 children aged 6 to 13 years conceived by in vitro fertilization. Fertil Steril 1997; 67: 284–9

44. Bradshaw J. Family Secrets: What You Don't Know Can Hurt You. London: Piatkus Books, 2001

45. Hoopes JL. Adoption and identity formation. In: Brodinsky DM, Scheter MD, eds. The Psychology of Adoption. Oxford: Oxford University Press, 1990: 144–66

46. Cook R, Vatev I, Michova Z, Golombok S. The European study of assisted reproduction families: a comparison of family functioning and child development between Eastern and Western Europe. J Psychosom Obstet Gynaecol 1997; 18: 203–12

47. Peters CJ, Kantaris X, Barnes J, Sutcliffe AG. Parental attitudes towards revealing mode of conception to their in-vitro fertilisation (IVF)-conceived child. Fertil Steril 2005; 83: 914–19

48. Cook R, Bradley S, Golombok S. A preliminary study of parental stress and child behaviour in families with twins conceived by in-vitro fertilization. Hum Reprod 1998; 13: 3244–6

49. Hay DA, McIndoe R, O'Brien PJ. The older siblings of twins. Aust J Early Child 1988; 13: 25–8

50. Bonduelle M, Wilikens A, Buysse A, et al. A follow-up study of children born after intracytoplasmic sperm injection (ICSI) with epididymal and testicular spermatozoa and after replacement of cryopreserved embryos obtained after ICSI. Hum Reprod 1998; 11: 1559–64

51. Bowen JR, Gibson FL, Leslie GI, Saunders DM. Medical and developmental outcome at 1 year for children conceived by intracytoplasmic sperm injection. Lancet 1998; 351: 1529–34

52. Gibson FL, Ungerer JA, McMahon C, et al. The mother–child relationship following in vitro fertilization (IVF): infant attachment, responsivity and maternal sensitivity. J Child Psychol Psychiatry 2000; 41: 1015–23

53. Golombok S, MacCallum F, Goodman E. The 'test-tube' generation: parent–child relationships and the psychological well-being of IVF children at adolescence. Child Dev 2001; 72: 599–608

54. Golombok S. Parenting and contemporary reproductive techniques. In: Bornstein MH, ed. Handbook of Parenting, vol 3. Mahwah, NJ: Lawrence Erlbaum Associates, 2002: 339–60

55. Munro J, Leeton J, Horsfall T. Psychosocial follow-up of families from a donor oocyte programme: an exploratory study. Reprod Fertil Dev 1992; 4: 125–30

56. Gibson FL, Ungerer JA, Tennant CC, Saunders DM. Parental adjustment and attitudes to parenting after in vitro fertilisation. Fertil Steril 2000; 73: 565–74

57. Weaver SM, Clifford E, Gordon AG, et al. A follow-up study of 'successful' IVF/GIFT couples: social-emotional well-being and adjustment to parenthood. J Psychosom Obstet Gynecol 1993; 14 (special issue): 5–16

58. Golombok S, Brewaeys A, Cook R, et al. The European study of assisted reproduction families: family functioning and child development. Hum Reprod 1996; 11: 2324–31

59. Golombok S, Murray C, Brinsden P, Abdulla H. Social versus biological parenting: family functioning and the socioemotional development of children conceived by egg or sperm donation. J Child Psychol Psychiatry 1999; 40: 519–27

60. Cook R, Golombok S, Bish A, Murray C. Keeping secrets: a study of parental attitudes toward telling about donor insemination. Am J Orthopsychiatry 1995; 65: 549–59

61. Golombok S, Brewaeys A, Giavazzi MT, et al. The European study of assisted reproduction families: the transition to adolescence. Hum Reprod 2002; 17: 830–40

62. Golombok S, MacCallum F. Practitioner review: outcomes for parents and children following non-traditional conception: what do clinicians need to know? J Child Psychol Psychiatry 2003; 44: 303–15

63. Barnes J, Sutcliffe AG, Kristoffersen I, et al. The influence of assisted reproduction on family functioning and children's socio-emotional development: results from a European study. Hum Reprod 2004; 19: 1480–7

64. Rohner RP. Handbook for the Study of Parental Acceptance and Rejection. Storrs, CT: University of Connecticut, 1999

65. Bene E. Manual for the Family Relations Test, 2nd edn. Slough, UK: NFER, 1985

66. Van Balen F. Child-rearing following in vitro fertilization. J Child Psychol Psychiatry 1996; 37: 687–93

67. Montgomery TR, Aiello F, Adelman D, et al. The psychological status at school age of children conceived by in-vitro fertilization. Hum Reprod 1999; 14: 2162–5

68. Gibson FL, Ungerer JA, Leslie GI, et al. Maternal attitudes to parenting and mother–child relationship and interaction in IVF families: a prospective study. Hum Reprod 1999; 14 (O238 Suppl 1): 131–2

69. Cederblad M, Friberg B, Ploman F, et al. Intelligence and behaviour in children born after in-vitro fertilization treatment. Hum Reprod 1996; 11: 2052–7

70. Soderstrom-Anttila V, Sajaniemi N, Tiitinen A, Hovatta O. Health and development of children born after oocyte donation compared with that of those born after in-vitro fertilization, and parents' attitudes regarding secrecy. Hum Reprod 1998; 13: 2009–15

71. Sutcliffe AG, Edwards PR, Beeson C, Barnes J. Comparing parents' perceptions of IVF conceived children's behaviour with naturally conceived children. Inf Mental Health J 2004; 25: 163–70

72. Kovacs GT, Mushin D, Kane H, Baker HWG. A controlled study of the psychosocial development of children conceived following insemination with donor semen. Hum Reprod 1993; 8: 788–90

73. Achenbach TM. Manual for the Child Behavior Checklist/4-18 and 1991 Profile. Burlington, VT: Department of Psychiatry, University of Vermont, 1991

74. McDevitt SC, Carey WB. The measurement of temperament in 3 to 7 year old children. J Child Psychol Psychiatry 1978; 19: 245–53

75. Abidin R. Parenting Stress Index Test Manual. Charlottesville, VA: Pediatric Psychology Press, 1990

76. Levy-Shiff R, Vakil E, Dimitrovsky L, et al. Medical, cognitive, emotional and behavioural outcomes in school-age children conceived by in-vitro fertilization. J Clin Child Psychol 1998; 27: 320–9

77. White J, Moffitt T, Earls F, et al. How early can we tell? Predictors of childhood conduct disorder and adolescent delinquency. Criminology 1990; 28: 507–33

78. Duncan S, Edwards R. Lone Mothers, Paid Work and Gendered Moral Rationalities. London: Macmillan, 1999

Chapter 7

Longer-term health of children conceived after ART – what we need to know

Alastair G Sutcliffe and Annika K Ludwig

The first edition of this book was given the title 'IVF Children: the First Generation'. This reflected on the fact that the oldest child who had been conceived by *in vitro* fertilization (IVF) was only 22 years old at the time of writing. A significant number of children whose parents had the benefit of them being conceived with the help of IVF are now in the teenage–early adult age range.

Some of them may be aware from time to time that issues are raised concerning their future health; often these issues are speculative but are nonetheless important. Ultimately, there are three core questions that will need to be addressed by research: future fertility; long-term risk of cancer; and risk of rare unexpected disorders such as imprintable disorders.

First and most obvious, fertility may be an issue for some of these children as they become adults, especially those males who have been conceived after the intracytoplasmic sperm injection (ICSI) type of assisted reproductive technology (ART). Here it is plausible to speculate that some of those grown men will have inherited from their fathers (where affected) Y chromosome deletions that had accounted for the male-factor infertility needing ICSI in their fathers.

The indications for ART appear to be widening and in my own lifetime as a doctor (AGS) the definition of infertility has been narrowed from 2 years with regular intercourse (where intercourse takes place two to three times per week) down to a year; as it has become recognized that if people do not conceive within a year they will be very unlikely to conceive naturally. As the use of ART has widened, the expense has fallen and the success rate risen; the number of people who are having borderline indications for ART has risen. Thus, whereas in the past the genetic and other risks to children born after ART in my view were higher, they have now probably fallen as the overall population of individuals having ART start to approach more closely the healthy population of naturally conceiving couples. Nonetheless, the child's future fertility will be a sensitive and relevant area of research.

Another area that will need to be investigated includes that surrounding the rare heritable disorders which are known as imprinting disorders. Here some research has been conducted highlighting the fact that there may be a problem for ART conception as a whole. These studies will be briefly described.

Third, another area which would be a critical outcome from ART is whether there is a higher risk of cancer in the offspring. Again, the known literature on this topic will be reviewed.

It is worthwhile taking a step back and considering how parents think when they have had an ART-conceived child and s/he develops an illness. Through the authors' privileged experiences of meeting and assessing over 700 children from different types of ART conception over a 10-year period, also speaking to many others on the telephone and indeed becoming aware of colleagues who have had IVF, a little insight into the mindset of some of these families has been obtained.

A postal survey of the families in the UK was conducted[1]. Approximately 500 families were contacted and they were divided approximately equally between naturally conceiving families, ICSI-conceiving families and IVF-conceiving families. This work, which was presented at the British Fertility Society (BFS) in April 2004, was fortunate to be recognized as the best abstract for counseling and psychosocial aspects of infertility and reproductive medicine. There were some key take-home messages from this and they are best illustrated by Figure 7.1, which shows the range of disorders that families thought might be due to ART conception. The families were particularly interested in whether the children would be fertile when they grew up. Many had no worries whatsoever. But there is a huge range of disorders that were enquired about in this postal survey. Many of these had little or no chance of being due to the mode of conception. However, this does give an insight for the practitioner about how families might think about such a major event as going through the process of having assisted conception. It may seem illogical but it also reflects the very nature of being a parent. One worries about one's children especially if they are ill, and one always searches for meaning even if that 'meaning' may be completely misguided. This also brings up a more important philosophical question which was asked astutely by one of the adjudicating team at the BFS presentation. Who would be responsible for the care implied by the concerns of these families?

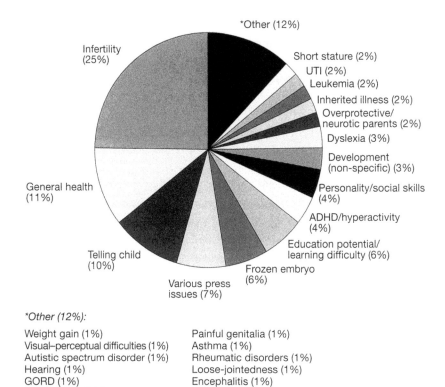

*Other (12%):

Weight gain (1%)
Visual–perceptual difficulties (1%)
Autistic spectrum disorder (1%)
Hearing (1%)
GORD (1%)
Food allergy (1%)
Chest problems (1%)

Painful genitalia (1%)
Asthma (1%)
Rheumatic disorders (1%)
Loose-jointedness (1%)
Encephalitis (1%)
Prematurity (1%)

Figure 7.1 Questions and concerns raised by families of ICSI/IVF children. ADHD, attention deficit/hyperactivity disorder; UTI, urinary tract infection; GORD, gastroesophageal reflux disease

There is no ideal answer, however, by acquiring more knowledge and insight into how families think at least one can be a little better prepared for these sorts of question. Families are often discreet and secretive, non-disclosing to most people about having had assisted conception, and thus would miss the opportunity to get answers to these anxiety-inducing questions. Perhaps the responsible initial person should be at the clinics which are providing treatment; counseling should be provided after the event and the family should be encouraged to come to see a counselor to discuss any issues.

The danger of handing this ongoing care over to uninformed individuals (concerning the literature surrounding outcome) is that they will give an inappropriate answer based on their own speculative curiosity. This may sound a little negative, but quite ignorant comments are often made about the dangers or not of ART conception to ART parents by medical colleagues in other specialties and in other anecdotal circumstances.

What can be said regarding the longer-term health of children born after ART that is not referred to in any of the other chapters of this book?

The literature search strategy is described in Chapter 6.

PHYSICAL HEALTH: CHILDHOOD AND CHRONIC ILLNESSES

Bonduelle *et al.* reported more childhood illnesses in children born after IVF or ICSI than after spontaneous conception[2]. Here the evidence was from the large ICSI–CFO study (see Chapter 6 for more details) and we speculated that this was due to increased parental concern rather than actual true increase. Similarly, Koivoruva *et al.* found that significantly more IVF children were diagnosed with at least one illness up to the age of 3 years. The cumulative incidence of respiratory disease, obstructive bronchitis or diarrhea requiring hospital treatment was increased in IVF singletons compared to spontaneously conceived singletons, while there was no difference for twins[3]. The difference in this study was likely to be due to the higher rates of premature birth. Other studies did not find a difference between IVF and spontaneously conceived children regarding childhood or chronic illnesses[2,4–11].

In a large cohort study including 9056 IVF children, Ericson *et al.*[12] reported that IVF children were more often hospitalized than spontaneously conceived children up to the age of 6 years. IVF children were significantly more frequently hospitalized for asthma or an infection. The odds ratio (OR) of being hospitalized after IVF was increased for singletons, twins and all infants born at term. Low maternal age, high parity, smoking and involuntary childlessness independently increased the risk of hospitalization. Most interestingly, the risk of being hospitalized increased with the duration of involuntary childlessness[12].

Some studies showed that the risk of being hospitalized and the number of days in hospital were increased for IVF twins compared to IVF singletons, but not compared to normally conceived twins[3,6,10,11]. Other studies did not show a difference between IVF and normally conceived children regarding hospital admissions[5,6,10], or ambulatory consultations of the pediatrician[7] or general practitioner[5], or routine visits to a child welfare center[9]. The Belgian group reported that physiotherapy and speech therapy were significantly more common in ICSI children compared to normally conceived children, while there was no difference regarding psychological therapy[4]. Wennerholm et al. found no difference regarding psychological therapy or therapy with a social welfare officer[9].

PHYSICAL EXAMINATION AND GROWTH

Malformations were not included in this chapter, as they are discussed by Ulla-Britt Wennerholm in her chapter. It is said that growth is a bioassay of wellbeing, and thus if a child's growth is satisfactory it is unlikely they are suffering from a serious ailment. None of the studies found differences in other aspects of the physical health of the children[2,13,14]. The incidence of vision or hearing impairment was not increased in IVF children in most studies[2,4,6]. Strömberg et al.[15] found more severe visual problems in IVF children than in the general population, although this increase was not statistically significant.

IVF and spontaneously conceived children did not differ regarding weight, height and head circumference[2,4,7,9,10,16,17] (Table 7.1)[2–18]. Only one group found IVF singletons to be lighter than the controls until the age of 3 years. In this study the IVF children were smaller in terms of weight and height at birth; catch-up growth was seen during the first year of life, but their growth was still behind that of the controls at the age of 3 years[3].

SURGICAL INTERVENTIONS

Some studies observed an increase in surgical interventions in singletons born after IVF or ICSI[2,4], while other studies showed no difference[7,10]. Bonduelle et al.[4] found that the higher rate of surgical interventions was mainly due to a higher rate of minor ear problems (tympanic drains, adenoidectomy). This could reflect differences in therapeutic attitude as well as a higher rate of recurrent infections or allergic conditions (see above). However, Bonduelle et al. did not find a higher incidence of infections that could have led to more surgical interventions[4].

In a prospective European multicenter study (the ICSI–CFO study) genitourinary surgery other than circumcision was more frequently performed in ICSI children than in spontaneously conceived children corresponding with a higher rate of genitourinary (GU) defects in boys conceived by ICSI[2]. This is perhaps unsurprising in view of the higher rate of GU defects in males needing ICSI.

There are only a few studies on twins. Pinborg et al. showed no difference regarding surgical interventions in IVF and SC twins aged 2–7 years, although IVF twins underwent significantly more surgical interventions

Table 7.1 Physical illnesses after ART

Author	Age	Cohorts	Illnesses and surgical interventions: other therapies	Physical examination and growth
Bonduelle et al., 2005[2]	4.5–5.5 years	540 ICSI singletons, 437 IVF singletons, 538 SC singletons Only Caucasian, ≥32 weeks of gestation, maternal or child language = national language, first or second born	More childhood illnesses in IVF and ICSI group: ICSI, 74%; IVF, 77%; SC, 57%; $p < 0.001$ More surgical intervention in IVF and ICSI group: ICSI, 24%; IVF, 22%; SC, 14%; $p < 0.001$ Genitourinary surgery other than circumcision: ICSI, 5%; IVF, 3%; SC, 1%; $p = 0.005$	No difference regarding physical examination No difference in hearing and vision No difference in height, weight, head circumference
Bonduelle et al., 2004[4]	5 years	300 ICSI singletons (100 Brussels, 98 Gottenberg, 102 New York), 266 SC singletons (100 Brussels, 111 Gottenberg, 55 New York) Only singletons, ≥32 weeks of gestation, maternal or child language = national language Only singletons, ≥32 weeks of gestation, no maternal or child language difference	No difference regarding chronic illnesses: ICSI, 8.0%; SC, 6.8% More surgical interventions in ICSI group: ICSI, 23%; SC, 16.5%; $p = 0.019$ Physiotherapy and speech therapy more common in ICSI group: Physiotherapy: ICSI, 2%; IVF, 1%; SC, 0; $p = 0.032$ Speech therapy: ICSI, 7%; IVF, 7%; SC, 4%; $p = 0.028$ No difference regarding psychological therapy	No difference regarding physical examination No difference in hearing and vision No difference in height, weight, head circumference

continued

Table 7.1 *Continued*

Author	Age	Cohorts	Illnesses and surgical interventions: other therapies	Physical examination and growth
Belva et al., 2004[18]	8 years	110 ICSI singletons, 109 SC singletons	No difference in number of hospital admissions, chronic diseases or behavioral problems	No difference in weight, height, head circumference No difference regarding physical examination No difference in pubertal development (Tanner scores)
Pinborg et al., 2004[11]	4 years (2–7 years)	3393 IVF/ICSI twins, 5139 IVF/ICSI singletons (all IVF/ICSI singletons and twins born in Denmark in 1995–2000), 10 239 SC (all SC twins born in Denmark in 1995–2000)	Frequency of hospitalization: IVF twins, 69.8%; SC twins, 69.6%; IVF singletons, 49.8%; OR adjusted for year of birth, maternal age, parity: IVF vs. SC twins: 1.00 (95% CI 0.91–1.11), OR IVF twins vs. IVF singletons: 2.38 (95% CI 2.17–2.63) Surgical interventions: IVF twins, 10.6%; SC twins, 11.2%; IVF singletons, 8.5% Adjusted OR IVF twins vs. singletons: 1.26 (95% CI 1.08–1.47), when only term infant: adjusted OR: 1.00 (95% CI 0.81–1.22)	

continued

Table 7.1 Continued

Author	Age	Cohorts	Illnesses and surgical interventions: other therapies	Physical examination and growth
			Average days in hospital: IVF twins, 14.5; SC twins, 13.8; IVF singletons, 5.3; IVF twins vs. singletons: $p < 0.001$ No differences in risk of admissions and surgical interventions for IVF vs. SC twins, for different sex IVF children and for IVF vs. ICSI twins	
Koivurova et al., 2003[3]	1–3, 4–9, 12, 18 months and 2, 3 years	1. 299 IVF children, 588 SC children (multiple birth rate 1.2% according to Finnish population) 2. 150 IVF singletons, 280 SC singletons 3. 100 IVF twins, 100 SC twins	More children with at least one diagnosed illness in IVF group: Full sample: OR 2.3 (95% CI 1.7–3.2), singletons: OR 2.1 (95% CI 1.3–3.3) Cumulative incidence of different disease requiring hospital treatment: IVF singletons, respiratory disease OR 3.1 (95% CI 1.0–9.4), obstructive bronchitis OR 5.1 (95% CI 1.3–19.1), diarrhea OR 5.7 (95% CI 2.6–12.7), twins: difference not significant	Full sample: IVF children shorter and lighter than controls up to 3 years Singletons: IVF children lighter than controls until the age of 3, height similar Twins: no difference

continued

Table 7.1 *Continued*

Author	Age	Cohorts	Illnesses and surgical interventions: other therapies	Physical examination and growth
Pinborg et al., 2003[6]	3–4 years	634 IVF or ICSI singletons and 1132 SC twins, 472 IVF or ICSI twins	No difference regarding common diseases, hospitalization (excluding neonatal care), number of admissions, ambulatory visits during last year, allergic disorders and chronic disorders (IVF twins, 16.1%; IVF singletons, 13.8%; SC twins,14.8%, NS) More surgical interventions in twins (IVF, 9.3%; SC, 8.7%) than in singletons (IVF, 5.8%; $p = 0.03$), IVF twins compared to IVF singletons: OR 1.7 (95% CI 1.1–2.6), difference disappeared after stratification for birth weight	No difference in hearing and vision
Place and Englert, 2003[7]	0–2 years, 3–5 years	66 ICSI singletons, 52 IVF singletons, 59 SC singletons Only full-term children, maternal age 20–40 years, one of the partners European, birth weight ≥ 2500 g, no conceptions in frozen–thawed cycles	No difference in minor or major health problems or the number of pediatric consultations No difference in minor surgical intervention	No difference in weight or height

continued

Table 7.1 *Continued*

Author	Age	Cohorts	Illnesses and surgical interventions: other therapies	Physical examination and growth
Ericson et al., 2002[12]	1–11 years	9056 IVF or ICSI children, 1 427 166 SC children	OR for being hospitalized after IVF increased up to age of 6 years: All children: OR 1.84 (95% CI 1.76–1.92) Singletons: OR 1.40 (95% CI 1.32–1.48) Twins: OR 1.17 (95% CI 1.07–1.27) All term infants: OR 1.34 (95% CI 1.27–1.41) Low maternal age, high parity, smoking, involuntary childlessness increased independently, risk of hospitalization OR for hospitalization for asthma or an infection significantly increased for IVF children Hospitalization in singletons, twins and children aged ≥6 years longer for IVF children	
Stromberg et al., 2002[15]	≥18 months	1. 5680 IVF children (3228 singletons) and 11 360 SC children (11 070 singletons) born 1982–1995 from the Swedish medical birth registry 2. 2060 IVF twins, 4120 SC twins		Severe visual disorders: OR 2.1 (95% CI 0.9–4.2) Only IVF multiples: OR 0.8 (95% CI 0.2–2.2) IVF singletons: OR 2.6 (95% CI 0.8–6.0)

continued

Table 7.1 *Continued*

Author	Age	Cohorts	Illnesses and surgical interventions: other therapies	Physical examination and growth
Bowen *et al.*, 1998[5]	13 months	89 ICSI children (69 singletons, 20 twins) 84 IVF children (55 singletons, 29 twins) 82 SC children (60 singletons, 20 twins)	No differences in incidence of hospital admissions, major health problems, visits to medical practitioner	No difference in height, weight, head circumference
Wennerholm *et al.*, 1998[9]	≤ 18 months	255 IVF children (fresh cycles) (160 singletons, 95 twins) 255 children from cryopreserved embryos (158 singletons, 97 twins), 252 SC children (156 singletons, 96 twins)	No difference in mean number of routine visits to child health center, chronic illnesses, atopy or common illnesses No differences regarding psychological therapy or therapy with social welfare officer	No difference in weight, height, head circumference or number of children with height 2 SD below mean length
Saunders *et al.*, 1996[10]	2 years	289 IVF children (196 singletons, 47 sets of twins, 8 sets of triplets), 146 SC children (114 singletons, 17 sets of twins, 1 set of triplets)	No differences regarding days in hospital post-initial discharge to age 2, and number of hospital admissions Twins had significantly more hospital admissions than singletons, males significantly more than females No difference regarding surgical interventions	No differences in weight, height and head circumference

continued

Table 7.1 *Continued*

Author	Age	Cohorts	Illnesses and surgical interventions: other therapies	Physical examination and growth
Raoul-Duval et al., 1994[8]	9, 18 months, 3 years	33 term-born IVF singletons, 33 term-born singletons after ovarian stimulation without IVF, 33 term-born SC singletons	Males had significantly more surgeries than females, due to circumcision, repair of inguinal herniae and hypospadias. No differences regarding infant illnesses, infant accidents, infant insomnia and feeding problems at 9 months, 18 months, 3 years	
Ron-El et al., 1994[14]	≥ 28 months	32 IVF singletons conceived after the use of GnRH-agonists, 32 SC singletons, born on the same day		No difference in physical examination
Brandes et al., 1992[16]	12–45 months	116 IVF children (66 singletons, 19 pairs of twins, 4 pairs of triplets), 116 SC children (66 singletons, 19 pairs of twins, 4 pairs of triplets)		No difference in weight, height and head circumference
Gershoni-Baruch et al., 1991[17]	13–20 months	33 IVF children (21 singletons, 12 twins) exposed to high-frequency transvaginal ultrasound (HFTS) in first trimester,		No difference in weight, height and head circumference

continued

Table 7.1 *Continued*

Author	Age	Cohorts	Illnesses and surgical interventions: other therapies	Physical examination and growth
		45 IVF children (29 singletons, 16 twins) not exposed, 33 SC children (21 singletons, 12 twins) exposed to HFTS, 45 SC children (29 singletons, 16 twins) not exposed		
Morin et al., 1989[13]	12–30 months	83 IVF children, 93 SC children		No differences in abdominal, cranial or cardiac ultrasound

ICSI, intracytoplasmic sperm injection; IVF, *in vitro* fertilization; SC, spontaneously conceived; NS, not significant; GnRH, gonadotropin releasing hormone compared to IVF singletons. However, this difference disappeared after adjustment for prematurity and birth weight[6,11,19].

BEHAVIOR

More detail is available on this topic in Professor Barnes' chapter. Only a few studies have concentrated on the child's socioemotional development. IVF children seem to develop well, as none of the studies found a difference between IVF and spontaneously conceived children regarding their behavior. In a rather small study of 27 IVF children and 23 spontaneously conceived children at the age of 8–9 years there was a trend towards more behavioral problems in IVF children reported by their teachers $(p = 0.06)$[20]. In another study significantly more IVF mothers (35%) than spontaneously conceived mothers (16%) felt that one of her 1-year-old child's behaviors was a problem for her. Overall, those studies that assessed children up to school age reported IVF children as having similar temperaments and similar levels of behavioral problems to the spontaneously conceived children.

CHILDHOOD CANCER

The issue of childhood cancer after assisted reproduction has been addressed in only a limited number of follow-up studies. The problem of analyzing this issue lies in the small incidence of childhood cancer. Therefore, large cohorts are essential for these studies. Some of the studies published so far have limited sample sizes for evaluating cancer risks; the larger studies generated the data on childhood cancer from national cancer registries. The number of IVF children included in the registry-based studies ranges from 2507[21] to 9479[22]. Two studies included only 176[23] and 332 IVF children[24], respectively, and therefore useful conclusions cannot be drawn[24]. Ideal sample size has been estimated to be at least 10 000 for most anomalies[25].

In the largest registry-based population-controlled study the number of expected cases reached 51 in 51 063 children[26], while most studies expected only 0–15 cases. In the largest study, a cohort of 30 364 Danish women were evaluated for infertility beginning in the early 1960s and therefore included children born after all types of infertility treatments[26].

None of the studies observed an increase in childhood cancer compared to all children born in the same time interval[6,11,12,19,27] or compared to expected incidence in the general population[21,24,26,28]. The control group of the study performed by Klip *et al.*[22] consisted of women with a history of subfertility who conceived spontaneously. The incidence of childhood cancer was also not increased in this study of 9478 children conceived after IVF, intrauterine insemination or ovulation induction[22].

These results are in contrast to a study by Moll et al.[29]. This group diagnosed a retinoblastoma in five patients born after IVF between November 2000 and February 2002. Assuming that these five cases represent all cases of retinoblastoma in children born after IVF, and estimating that in The Netherlands 1.0–1.5% of children are born after IVF the authors calculated that 0.69 retinoblastoma cases would be expected in children conceived after IVF between 1995 and 2001. Based on this assumption they calculated a significantly increased risk ratio of 7.2 (95% CI 2.4–17.0)[29]. However, this study has been widely discussed. It has been questioned whether these five cases might be a clustering detected by an 'interested' observer. If, in the period studied by Moll et al.[29], 3.0% instead of 1.0–1.5% of live births in The Netherlands were conceived after ART, the relative risk for retinoblastoma would be much lower than the reported risk of 4.9 for 1.5% (95% CI 1.6–11.3) and 7.2 for 1.0% (95% CI 2.4–17.0)[30]. Furthermore, attention has to be paid to the very wide confidence intervals in the study by Moll et al.

A few case–control studies have suggested an increased risk of neuroblastoma[31,32] and leukemia[33,34] in the children of women treated with infertility drugs. The epidemiology of neuroblastoma suggests that prenatal drug exposures may be important etiological factors in the disease. However, larger cohort studies among IVF children have not shown an increased risk of neuroblastoma or leukemia compared with the general population to date[22,27,28].

Overall, this question is unresolved. Alastair Sutcliffe is currently conducting a national study of retinoblastoma to establish whether there is a higher risk following ART conception. Other studies are ongoing which may finally link the British Human Fertilisation and Embryology Authority (HFEA) database with the British Childhood Cancer Registry, allowing us to investigate whether there is any risk from ART. It would seem from the above evidence that there is insufficient information to decide whether there is a higher risk to these children. Most human cancers develop over a period of 20 years before they manifest (Professor Tim Oliver, Professor of Oncology at London University, personal communication) and thus this question will still remain unresolved for some time.

IMPRINTING DISORDERS AND ART

Finally we comment on the emerging evidence that imprintable disorders are more common after assisted conception. Genomic imprinting is the mechanism that determines the expression or repression of genes from maternal or paternal chromosomes. This modification of genetic material is epigenetic, i.e. reversible between generations, and is not a mutation. Maternal and paternal germlines confer an imprint or sex-specific mark on certain chromosome regions. Therefore, although the sequence of the genes on these chromosomes could be identical, they are not functionally equivalent.

Over 40 imprinted genes have now been characterized. They have been shown to influence embryonic growth and development and are implicated in the inactivation of tumor suppressor genes, resulting in some childhood cancers, e.g. Wilms' tumor, embryonal rhabdomyosarcoma, osteosarcoma and bilateral retinoblastoma. These are thought to occur by the 'two-hit' hypothesis of cancer. The first inactivation of a tumor suppressor allele would occur by imprinting rather than by mutation. Wilms' tumor appears to have two different tumor precursor lesions. One type is thought to be due to an imprinting defect of the gene for insulin-like growth factor-II (IGF-II). The second subtype occurs after a mutation of the *WT1* gene.

There is evidence that several syndromes are also caused by imprinting disorders, such as Prader–Willi syndrome, Angelman syndrome, Russell–Silver syndrome, transient neonatal diabetes, Beckwith–Wiedemann syndrome, pseudohypoparathyroidism and McCune–Albright syndrome. In a nutshell, in ART, concern exists that a gene not ordinarily expressed (i.e. imprinted) undergoes unscheduled expression. This could reflect underlying parental characteristics or *in vitro* culture changes.

The first child (a boy) to be recorded in the medical literature who had Beckwith–Wiedemann syndrome and who was also born after embryo cryopreservation[35] was about 5 years of age and was remarkably well. Beckwith–Wiedemann syndrome is a variable condition, which ranges from being moderately to mildly significant in a child's life, assuming they do not acquire a complication from it. In this little boy, you would never have guessed he had anything wrong with him. Nonetheless, having left the consultation, the editor frivolously remarked that he had discovered the cause of Beckwith–Wiedemann syndrome, which was embryo cryopreservation! Little did one know that some 10 years later there would be evidence emerging that there may be a higher risk of imprintable disorders after ART.

Two case–control studies have shown an association between ART and Beckwith–Wiedemann syndrome[36,37]. Beckwith–Wiedemann syndrome is an overgrowth disorder characterized by macrosomia, macroglossia, omphalocele and embryonal cancer. Case reports describe other imprinting disorders that have occurred after ART. DeBaun *et al.*[38] conducted a case–control study of Beckwith–Wiedemann registry cases, finding that three of 65 cases had undergone ART. Molecular studies of these three as well as two other cases showed five of six to have unexpected maternal expression of the imprinted *BWS* gene. Moreover, this is an uncommon molecular explanation for Beckwith–Wiedemann syndrome. That overexpression occurs in an overgrowth disorder such as Beckwith–Wiedemann syndrome is intriguing. Similar findings were made in a UK study by Maher *et al.*[39], using a UK Beckwith–Wiedemann syndrome registry. Of 149 children with the syndrome, six (4%) had been the product of ART – three IVF alone and three ICSI plus IVF. Furthermore, it has been known for many years that monozygotic (MZ) twinning is also increased after ART and the genetic mechanism for MZ twinning (still not fully understood) appears also to be implicated in Beckwith–Wiedemann syndrome (namely via overexpression of the *IGF2* gene).

More recent studies have tempered concern. Chang *et al.*[40] studied 12 Beckwith–Wiedemann children who were the products of IVF or ICSI; no common factor was observed with respect to ovulation stimulation or tissue culture. Ludwig *et al.*[41] studied the imprinting disorder Angelman syndrome, and found that among 16 cases four were born to *subfertile* couples. The four did not require ART; however, their time to conception exceeded 2 years or they required hormonal stimulation. This is another example of an infertile sample differing from the general population; the perturbation responsible for the infertility could well predispose offspring to disorders of imprinting. Another relevant dataset was derived from the Danish IVF registry[42], which was cross-linked with other registries to search for disorders known or thought to be related to imprinting. Those queried were Beckwith–Wiedemann, Prader–Willi and Angleman syndromes. A total of 442 349 singleton non-IVF pregnancies were compared to 605 IVF pregnancies with offspring born during 1995–2002. Disorders sought were proved or thought potentially to be related to imprinting: Beckwith–Wiedemann syndrome, Prader–Willi syndrome, Angelman syndrome and, more speculatively, cancer, mental retardation and cerebral palsy. Only in the cerebral palsy group did the imprinting disorders associated with IVF exceed those that did not.

So, what can be concluded about the overall future health of ART-conceived children? First, in this chapter, it can be reasonably stated that there appears to be a slightly higher risk of medical illnesses and surgical interventions in this population of children. Whether this is a true effect, or a result of increased parental concern, remains to be confirmed. Furthermore, the surgical interventions may reflect the now well recognized risk of congenital anomalies which, albeit only slightly above that of the naturally conceived population of children, is still slightly increased on the background. Second, there do not appear to be any specific behavioral problems related to being an ART-conceived child on the basis of studies so far, but these are few, and children would need to be studied at an older age. Finally, there are outstanding issues concerning the children's future fertility, which will be a very difficult issue to investigate. Furthermore, there is an emerging field of evidence suggesting that there might be an increased risk of imprintable disorders after ART conception, probably as a result of the couples' history of infertility, rather than of the procedures themselves.

REFERENCES

1. Fisher-Jeffes LJ, Banerjee I, Sutcliffe AG. Parents' concerns regarding their ART children. Reproduction 2006; 131: 389–94
2. Bonduelle M, Wennerholm UB, Loft A, et al. A multi-centre cohort study of the physical health of 5-year-old children conceived after intracytoplasmic sperm injection, in vitro fertilization and natural conception. Hum Reprod 2005; 20: 413–19
3. Koivurova S, Hartikainen AL, Sovio U, et al. Growth, psychomotor development and morbidity up to 3 years of age in children born after IVF. Hum Reprod 2003; 18: 2328–36
4. Bonduelle M, Bergh C, Niklasson A, et al. Medical follow-up study of 5-year-old ICSI children. Reprod Biomed Online 2004; 9: 91–101
5. Bowen JR, Gibson FL, Leslie GI, Saunders DM. Medical and developmental outcome at 1 year for children conceived by intracytoplasmic sperm injection. Lancet 1998; 351: 1529–34
6. Pinborg A, Loft A, Schmidt L, Andersen AN. Morbidity in a Danish national cohort of 472 IVF/ICSI twins, 1132 non-IVF/ICSI twins and 634 IVF/ICSI singletons: health-related and social implications for the children and their families. Hum Reprod 2003; 18: 1234–43
7. Place I, Englert Y. A prospective longitudinal study of the physical, psychomotor, and intellectual development of singleton children up to 5 years who were conceived by intracytoplasmic sperm injection compared with children conceived spontaneously and by in vitro fertilization. Fertil Steril 2003; 80: 1388–97
8. Raoul-Duval A, Bertrand-Servais M, Letur-Konirsch H, Frydman R. Psychological follow-up of children born after in-vitro fertilization. Hum Reprod 1994; 9: 1097–101
9. Wennerholm UB, Albertsson-Wikland K, Bergh C, et al. Postnatal growth and health in children born after cryopreservation as embryos. Lancet 1998; 351: 1085–90
10. Saunders K, Spensley J, Munro J, Halasz G. Growth and physical outcome of children conceived by in vitro fertilization. Pediatrics 1996; 97: 688–92

11. Pinborg A, Loft A, Rasmussen S, Nyboe Andersen A. Hospital care utilization of IVF/ICSI twins followed until 2–7 years of age: a controlled Danish national cohort study. Hum Reprod 2004; 19: 2529–36

12. Ericson A, Nygren KG, Olausson PO, Kallen B. Hospital care utilization of infants born after IVF. Hum Reprod 2002; 17: 929–32

13. Morin NC, Wirth FH, Johnson DH, et al. Congenital malformations and psychosocial development in children conceived by in vitro fertilization. J Pediatr 1989; 115: 222–7

14. Ron-El R, Lahat E, Golan A, et al. Development of children born after ovarian superovulation induced by long-acting gonadotropin-releasing hormone agonist and menotropins, and by in vitro fertilization. J Pediatr 1994; 125: 734–7

15. Stromberg B, Dahlquist G, Ericson A, et al. Neurological sequelae in children born after in-vitro fertilisation: a population-based study. Lancet 2002; 359: 461–5

16. Brandes JM, Scher A, Itzkovits J, et al. Growth and development of children conceived by in vitro fertilization. Pediatrics 1992; 90: 424–9

17. Gershoni-Baruch R, Scher A, Itskovitz J, et al. The physical and psychomotor development of children conceived by IVF and exposed to high-frequency vaginal ultrasonography (6.5 MHz) in the first trimester of pregnancy. Ultrasound Obstet Gynecol 1991; 1: 21–8

18. Belva F, Boelaert K, Leunens L, et al. Medical outcomes of eight year old ICSI children. Hum Reprod 2004; 19: abstr I112

19. Pinborg A, Loft A, Schmidt L, et al. Neurological sequelae in twins born after assisted conception: controlled national cohort study. Br Med J 2004; 329: 311

20. Colpin H, Soenen S. Parenting and psychosocial development of IVF children: a follow-up study. Hum Reprod 2002; 17: 1116–23

21. Doyle P, Bunch KJ, Beral V, Draper GJ. Cancer incidence in children conceived with assisted reproduction technology. Lancet 1998; 352: 452–3

22. Klip H, Burger CW, de Kraker J, van Leeuwen FE. Risk of cancer in the offspring of women who underwent ovarian stimulation for IVF. Hum Reprod 2001; 16: 2451–8

23. Bradbury BD, Jick H. In vitro fertilization and childhood retinoblastoma. Br J Clin Pharmacol 2004; 58: 209–11

24. Lerner-Geva L, Toren A, Chetrit A, et al. The risk for cancer among children of women who underwent in vitro fertilization. Cancer 2000; 88: 2845–7

25. Sutcliffe AG. IVF Children: the First Generation. Assisted Reproduction and Child Development, 1st edn. London: Parthenon Publishing, 2002

26. Brinton LA, Kruger KS, Thomsen BL, et al. Childhood tumor risk after treatment with ovulation-stimulating drugs. Fertil Steril 2004; 81: 1083–91

27. Bergh T, Ericson A, Hillensjo T, et al. Deliveries and children born after in-vitro fertilisation in Sweden 1982–95: a retrospective cohort study [see comments]. Lancet 1999; 354: 1579–85

28. Bruinsma F, Venn A, Lancaster P, et al. Incidence of cancer in children born after in-vitro fertilization. Hum Reprod 2000; 15: 604–7

29. Moll AC, Imhof SM, Cruysberg JR, et al. Incidence of retinoblastoma in children born after in-vitro fertilisation. Lancet 2003; 361: 309–10

30. BenEzra D. In vitro fertilisation and retinoblastoma. Lancet 2003; 361: 273–4

31. Kramer S, Ward E, Meadows AT. Medical drug risk factors associated with neuroblastoma: a case–control study. J Natl Cancer Inst 1987; 78: 797–804

32. Michalek AM, Buck GM, Nasca PC. Gravid health status, medication use, and risk of neuroblastoma. Am J Epidemiol 1996; 143: 996–1001

33. Roman E, Ansell P, Bull D. Leukaemia and non-Hodgkin's lymphoma in children and young adults: are prenatal and neonatal factors important determinants of disease? Br J Cancer 1997; 76: 406–35

34. Steensel-Moll HA, Valkenburg HA, Vanderbroucke JP. Are maternal fertility problems related to childhood leukaemia? J Epidemiol 1985; 14: 555–9

35. Sutcliffe AG, DeSouza SW, Cadman J, et al. Minor congenital anomalies, major congenital malformations and development in children conceived from cryopreserved embryos. Hum Reprod 1995; 10: 3332–7

36. Cox GF, Burger J, Lip V, et al. Intracytoplasmic sperm injection may increase risks of imprinting defects. Am J Hum Genet 2002; 71: 162–4

37. Gicquel C, Gaston V, Mandelbaum J, et al. In vitro fertilisation may increase risk of Beckwith–Wiedemann syndrome related to the abnormal imprinting of the KCN1OT gene. Am J Hum Genet 2003; 72: 1338–41

38. DeBaun MR, Niemitz EL, Feinberg AP. Association of in vitro fertilization with Beckwith–Wiedemann syndrome and epigenetic alterations of LIT1 and H19. Am J Hum Genet 2003; 72: 156–60

39. Maher ER, Brueton LA, Bowdin SC, et al. Beckwith–Wiedemann syndrome and assisted reproductive technology (ART). J Med Genet 2003; 40: 62–4

40. Chang AS, Moley KH, Wangler M, et al. Association between Beckwith–Wiedemann syndrome and assisted reproductive technology: a case series of 19 patients. Fertil Steril 2005; 83: 349–54

41. Ludwig M, Katalinic A, Gross S, et al. Increased prevalence of imprinting defects in patients with Angelman syndrome born to subfertile couples. J Med Genet 2005; 42: 289–91

42. Lidegaard O, Pinborg A, Andersen AN. Imprinting diseases and IVF: Danish National IVF cohort study. Hum Reprod 2005; 20: 950–4

Chapter 8

Special considerations of twin and higher-order births

Elizabeth Bryan and Jane Denton

When Louise Brown was born in 1978, there was widespread anxiety about the risks and implications of *in vitro* fertilization (IVF) but few expected what has proved to be the greatest risk, that of an epidemic of multiple pregnancies. Even now it appears that there are many couples embarking on treatment for their infertility who are unaware of the risks and implications of a multiple pregnancy let alone what is entailed in the care and upbringing of multiple-birth children. Many imagine that twins would be an ideal outcome and some may well believe they would be fortunate to have triplets: an instant family.

Unfortunately, too few studies have assessed the problems multiples can present. Many of the studies on IVF outcomes have either excluded twins or failed to distinguish them from the singleborn. In view of the very different pregnancy, perinatal and parenting experiences of these families, a separate chapter on the implications of a multiple pregnancy is all too justified.

EPIDEMIOLOGY – INTERNATIONAL OVERVIEW

Throughout the developed world there has been a steady rise in the incidence of twin births since the early 1980s[1-3]. In England and Wales it has risen from 9.8 per thousand births in 1980 to 14.61 in 2003[4] (Figure 8.1). In 2000 the rates in Europe ranged from 10.55 in Luxembourg to 20.05 in Greece[3].

The incidence of triplets in England and Wales rose still faster until 1998, quadrupling in 15 years. It has now started to decline again[4] (Figure 8.2).

Other countries have had an even more dramatic rise[3] with a triplet rate of 0.7 in Spain compared to 0.44 in the UK and 0.2 in Sweden.

These increases in multiple births are known to be largely due to the widespread use in the treatment of subfertility of inadequately monitored ovulation induction and multiple embryo transfer[5,6]. Israel, the country with the highest number of IVF cycles per head of population in the world, has also had the most rapid rise in its twinning rate[7]. An additional

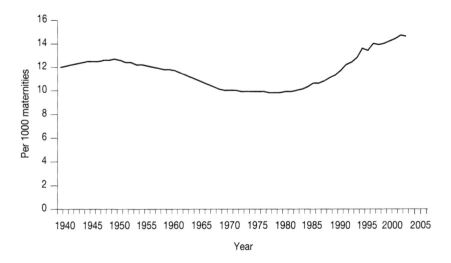

Figure 8.1 Twinning rate in England and Wales 1940–2003. From reference 4

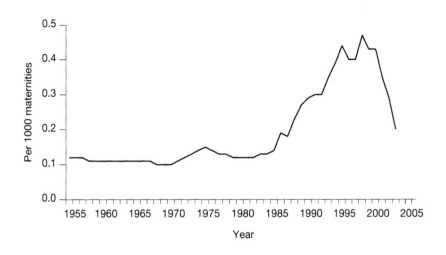

Figure 8.2 Triplet rate in England and Wales 1955–2003. From reference 4

factor in the rising twinning rate has been the increase in average maternal age[2] as women delay childbearing. Spontaneous twinning is known to increase with maternal age until the late thirties[8].

East Flanders in Belgium is the only region that has so far provided accurate population-based data on the origin of all multiple births, including ovulation induction, and has done so since 1964[9]. In most countries accurate data on conception are only available for those multiple births that arise following IVF or gamete donation. The most recent figures from the UK's Human Fertilisation and Embryology Authority reported 24.1% of multiple births following IVF in 2003 – of which 0.5% were triplets and 23.6% twins[10].

Since reducing the numbers of embryos transferred to two in the early 1990s, Sweden has seen a fall in twinning rate following IVF from 29% in 1991 to 18.5% in 2001. A further fall is expected following the recently introduced policy of single embryo transfer[11].

Most of the resulting multiple pregnancies following ovulation induction and multiembryo transfer are multizygotic. It is the increase in dizygotic (DZ) twinning that is largely responsible for the current upward trends in twinning. Although DZ twinning rates vary greatly in different parts of the world[12], the trends are similar wherever new techniques in treatment for infertility are practiced. In general, races of black African origin have the highest rates of DZ twins; the Far Eastern races have the lowest; the rates for Asian Indians and Caucasians lie between.

ZYGOSITY

There are clear medical and scientific reasons for determining zygosity[13] in addition to the parents' wish to know[13,14]. Although obstetricians now appreciate the importance of determining the chorionicity in a multiple pregnancy, some appear to be less concerned with the accurate determination of zygosity. Indeed, there are many, even now, who continue to misinform parents by telling them that their twins are definitely DZ because they have a dichorionic placenta[15], despite the well-established fact that about one-third of monozygotic (MZ) twins also have dichorionic placentae.

For an infertile couple an essential part of their pretreatment counseling is information on the true incidence of MZ twinning following ovulation induction or assisted reproductive technology (ART) as well as the implications of a monochorionic placenta. A single embryo transfer that results in twins can clearly be most disconcerting for a couple. When a two-embryo transfer results in triplets, parents may be seriously upset.

Furthermore, a monochorionic placenta carries additional risks for the fetuses due to the shared fetal circulation and consequent risk of hemodynamic imbalance. The twin–twin transfusion syndrome occurs in 10–15% of monochorionic pregnancies[16] and is associated with a high perinatal mortality rate and a substantial risk of long-term neurological morbidity[17–19].

Until recently, and unlike DZ twinning, the prevalence of MZ twin births had remained constant worldwide at 3.5 per 1000 maternities. Since the early 1990s there has been a small increase[12]. Although the majority of iatrogenic twins are DZ, there appears to be a higher than expected incidence of MZ twinning following ovulation induction with or without embryo transfer. In the East Flanders Prospective Twin Study 11.4% of iatrogenic triplets included an MZ pair[20]. Amongst iatrogenic twins overall, the rate was 10 times that of spontaneous conceptions. With ovulation induction it was 14 times.

As very few infertility or maternity units routinely determine zygosity, as opposed to chorionicity, estimates of the frequency of MZ splitting depend on various indirect methods of assessment, which have their own inherent problems[21]. Counting the number of monochorionic twins will underestimate the frequency of MZ twins, as those with dichorionic placentas will be missed. Furthermore, it has still to be determined whether the proportion of MZ twins with a dichorionic placenta is the same, i.e. one-third, amongst iatrogenic MZ twins as in those conceived spontaneously.

It might be expected that there would be a higher incidence of monochorionic twins amongst pregnancies arising from blastocyst transfer because their transfer, unlike the 3-day embryo transfer, happens when the placental mass is already forming and a split would therefore result in a higher proportion of monochorionic twins. In a 3-day embryo any split would be expected to result in a dichorionic pair. It has also been suggested that, in the case of the blastocyst where there has been a longer extrauterine period, the zona pellucida may have been at greater risk of damage. Several studies have shown such an increase in MZ splitting[22].

MZ twinning rates can also be estimated using Weinberg's differential rule. This states that the number of MZ twins is estimated by calculating the sum total of DZ twins in a population as twice the number of unlike-sexed twins and subtracting this sum from the total. However, this may not be satisfactory, as this rule depends on there being equal numbers of male and female twins. It has been suggested that the male/female ratio may differ between spontaneously and iatrogenically conceived twins and between different stages of transfer. Combining the results of seven studies, Milki and colleagues[23] found that the proportion of males was 57.3% in the blastocyst transfers compared to 51.2% in 3-day embryo transfers.

Finally, estimates of MZ splitting have been made by studying the number of single embryo transfers that result in a twin pregnancy and of two-embryo transfer resulting in triplets (although the rare occurrence of superfecundation cannot be excluded, the transferred embryo then being accompanied by a spontaneous conception).

The only population-based study of single embryo transfer in relation to monozygosity was carried out in a British population at a time when few, if any, of the single embryo transfers were elective[24]. In the great majority of cases they were performed because only one embryo was available. In this group there was a three-fold increase in MZ splitting. However, the incidence of splitting in single high-quality embryos transferred electively may be different.

The only reliable estimation of MZ splitting rates must be through routine zygosity determination. To date, East Flanders is the only population in which this has been comprehensively carried out. The figures there suggest that about 5–7% of all iatrogenic twins are MZ[20].

Findings of increases in the incidence of MZ splitting are consistent, although the frequency varies. The reason for this high splitting rate is unknown, as are the factors causing MZ twinning in general. Hormone treatment, the less than optimum intrauterine environment of some subfertile women, micromanipulation of the embryo and the *in vitro* culture medium have all been suggested as triggers to MZ twinning in iatrogenic pregnancies. The varying factors, as well as the form of estimation, may affect the recorded incidence of MZ twinning within a particular population.

Very recently a new phenomenon has been reported – that of monochorionic dizygotic twinning following ART[25]. Miura and Niikawa[25] reported six cases from Japan and suggested that it was due to fusion between the outer cell masses from two adjacent zygotes and that this fusion may be facilitated by changes in the nature of the cell surface caused by factors such as assisted hatching, blastocyst stage embryos and *in vitro* cell culture. It remains to be seen how often this placentation occurs following ART. In spontaneous human twinning the situation is extremely rare[20]. Chimerism occurs due to the shared intrauterine blood circulation, but there have as yet been no reports of the 'freemartin' effect seen in other species, such as cattle, with suppression of female genital development resulting from raised levels of male hormones in the female fetus.

THE IMPLICATIONS OF MULTIPLE BIRTHS

Multiple births are increasingly large contributors to the preterm and low-birth-weight population in most developed countries. The average duration of pregnancy for twins in the UK is 37 weeks, 33.5 for triplets and 31.5 for quadruplets[26], and a little lower in the USA[27]. About half of twins, over 90% of triplets and nearly all quadruplets are born preterm (< 37 weeks) compared to 10% of singletons[27].

The average weight of a newborn twin is about 800 g less than that of a singleton[28]. Fifty per cent of twins, 90% of triplets and nearly all quadruplets have a birth weight of less than 2500 g, compared with 6% of singletons. As many as 10% of twins, 32% of triplets and over half the quadruplets weigh less than 1500 g[29]. Indeed, twins and triplets contributed at least 35% of the very low birth weight (VLBW) infants in a population-based study from Israel[29].

It has been repeatedly shown that IVF singleborn children are at greater risk than spontaneously conceived singletons in terms of prematurity, low birth weight and neonatal complications. Twins are at these disadvantages to a much greater extent compared to singleborn children. However, the difference between IVF twins and spontaneously conceived twins appears to be less than that between the two singleborn groups[30,31].

It may well be that the difference in zygosity distribution between iatrogenic and spontaneously conceived twins counteracts the disadvantages imposed by induced pregnancies. As a higher proportion of iatrogenic twins are DZ than amongst twins who are spontaneously conceived, the iatrogenic twins in general would be expected to fare better. There is little evidence of this.

Only one study has shown iatrogenic twins to be advantaged[32] and in this case the higher perinatal mortality rate in the spontaneously conceived group was attributed to the complications of monochorionicity. Some have found no difference[33,34] but the majority have found the ART twins to be at a disadvantage in terms of prematurity[35–37], low birth weight[35–38], higher cesarean section rate[37], length of stay in the neonatal intensive care unit[37] and perinatal mortality[35,36,39]. The one study that controlled for zygosity by limiting the study to DZ twins found that ART twins had a small but significant reduction in gestational age and birth weight and a higher perinatal mortality rate[35].

Inevitably most if not all these studies will have other biases. For instance, few have allowed for the highly significant confounding variables of maternal age, parity and socioeconomic status.

Later development of multiple-birth children

Owing primarily to the complications of preterm delivery and low birth weight, multiple-birth children are likely to suffer more health problems in the early years[40] and are at much greater risk than singletons of long-term neurodevelopmental disorders, particularly cerebral palsy.

Population studies have shown a three- to seven-fold higher incidence of cerebral palsy in twins compared to singletons and one over ten-fold higher in triplets[41,42]. The highest rate of cerebral palsy is in surviving children whose co-twin or triplet died *in utero*[41,43]. The chances of any particular multiple pregnancy producing a bereaved family or a disabled child are of course much greater still[41,44].

In a multicenter population-based study from 12 European countries Topp and colleagues[42] found a four-fold increase in cerebral palsy amongst multiples with 56% of those affected being secondborn. Unlike IVF singletons, there is little evidence that these problems are any greater amongst IVF- than spontaneously conceived twins, although the growth, health and neurodevelopment of all twins is worse than for singletons[30,40,45].

Higher-order births

It is universally recognized that the greater the number of fetuses, the greater the risk of maternal complications during the pregnancy, the slower the growth of each fetus and the higher the rate of preterm delivery, neonatal complications, perinatal mortality and long-term neurodisability.

There are, however, some aspects of a triplet pregnancy that are surprising. Unlike singletons, the offspring of older mothers appear, if anything, to be at an advantage[46,47]. This may well be because most of these older mothers conceived triplets following IVF and therefore are likely to come from high socioeconomic groups with access to the best obstetric and neonatal care.

However great the improvement in long-term outcome of these higher multiples following the recent progress in neonatal care, triplets will always be at a disadvantage to singletons. Their conception through ART should never be regarded in a positive light. Furthermore, the great majority of their parents suffer from physical and emotional stress as well as, in many cases, considerable financial hardship[26,48,49].

Psychosocial issues

Contrary to the expectations of many couples that twins or triplets would be an ideal outcome of their infertility treatment, the realities of a multiple pregnancy can come as quite a shock.

Parenting

A multiple pregnancy is more likely to be associated with medical complications such as hypertensive disorders including pre-eclampsia, anemia, polyhydramnios, preterm labor and a difficult delivery. In addition, the mother is likely to suffer from tiredness, indigestion and general discomfort far earlier than with a single baby. Following a multiple pregnancy a mother is therefore often ill prepared for the physical and emotional stresses of caring for two or more babies at the same time. Mothers of twins have been shown to suffer more from lack of sleep and fatigue than mothers of a singleborn[50] and this may be a particular problem for the increasing number of older mothers. Mothers of multiples, whether or not they have had infertility problems, also have a higher risk of depression in the early years[51]. Isolation and fatigue are probably both significant contributory factors to this. Furthermore, the mothers are likely to have babies who are more vulnerable and difficult to care for. Not surprisingly, child abuse has been shown to be more common in multiple birth families with the disadvantaged of the two children being the more likely to be affected[52].

With two babies a mother may be frustrated by her inability to give each baby the attention they need and this reduction in interaction on her part has been shown to effect the cognitive development of the children at 18 months[53]. Similarly, with triplets it was shown that they were at risk of delay in cognitive development, at least during the first 2 years and that this was related in part to the difficulty of providing sensitive mothering to three infants at the same time[54].

Feldman and Eidelman[54] also found that when there was birth-weight discordancy within the set, the smallest triplet tended to do less well and to receive less positive attention from the mother. Similarly, the disadvantage for the smaller infant in mother–infant relationships has been seen in twins[55].

The mother's stress may be reinforced by the attitude of other people. The parents may be made to feel stigmatized by their infertility. When seen with their twin children, let alone triplets, they may receive intrusive and unwelcome comments, even jokes, making the parents feel vulnerable to public evaluation of their fertility status[26,56,57] (Box 8.1).

For those whose children arrive after many years of uncertainty and having dreamt of the perfect child, the stresses of two or three vulnerable babies will be even greater. The emotional challenges of infertility can deplete the psychological resources of women and to some extent of their partners[58]. When pregnancy finally comes, many, particularly those who have become depressed by the treatment, have insufficient time to restore their psychological reserves before they are faced with the transition to

---

Box 8.1

Comments by strangers to mothers of triplets

"I don't mean to be personal but are they yours or did you have fertility treatment?"

"How will you cope?"

"Are they test tube ones?"

Botting BJ, MacFarlane AJ, Price FV, eds. *Three, Four and More. A Study of Triplet and Higher Order Births.* London: HMSO, 1990

---

parenthood. If there are added and often unexpected stresses or anxieties, as inevitably arise in a multiple pregnancy, mothers are likely to be at higher risk of postpartum depression[59].

Studies of singleborn children have shown that both parent satisfaction and parenting skills with IVF children are, if anything, superior to those with spontaneously conceived children, but the situation may be different with twins. Glazebrook and colleagues[60] compared two groups of first-time mothers who had conceived after IVF treatment: one with twins and the other with singleborns: 22% of mothers of twins suffered from severe parenting stress compared to 5% with singleborn children. Pinborg et al.[61] found that the parenting and marital stress for all parents of twins was greater than with the singleborn but there was no difference between those with iatrogenic twins than those with spontaneously conceived twins.

In a small study comparing 12 families with 4–8-year-old IVF twins and 14 with spontaneously conceived twins, Cook et al.[62] found that parenting stress for both mothers and fathers was greater in the IVF group. Although the quality of parenting was equally good, parental satisfaction was less. This could well be due to the parents' inevitable failure to reach the high standards of parenting they had set themselves and had for so long expected to achieve[63].

Furthermore, Munro et al.[64] found that IVF families with preschool-age twins tended to have poorer social support. Again, they may have become isolated during their long quest for a child and then found themselves both older and of a different lifestyle than many of the parents of their young children's friends. The situation is, however, likely to vary in different settings and cultures. In Belgium, Colpin et al.[65] found no difference in parenting stress or psychosocial wellbeing within the two groups.

The first population-based study of the psychosocial outcome for families with twins, which therefore avoided the biases resulting from families being chosen from specific infertility clinics, was recently reported by Tully and colleagues[66]. They found that IVF and ovulation induction (OI) families were functioning well and no less well than those that had spontaneously conceived offspring. In fact, the IVF/OI couples tended to agree with each other more and had more similar parenting styles. There was no difference in child behavior.

The outcomes for parents, and the warmth shown towards their children, were similar to those found in the non-IVF/OI group. Nevertheless, they did not show the degree of enhanced warmth that was seen in the parents of IVF singleborn children.

The care of a child with special needs always brings challenges for parents. In multiple-birth families these are increased by the difficulty of caring for other children of the same age, but with very different needs[67].

Added stresses may result from bereavement[68]. During the neonatal period parents who lose one of their babies have the emotional ambivalence of grieving for the death of one child whilst celebrating the life of the other. Too often they may have agonizing weeks watching their very preterm infants struggling to survive. Later they may have to cope with the emotional problems of the surviving twin or triplet whilst having a constant reminder in them of the child who died[69].

Even for those parents who end up with two healthy children, there may still be an unexpected sense of loss. For those who go through long years of infertility treatment they can be distressed by the frustration of not being able to give each baby the time and undivided attention they had always envisaged. In our experience there are many mothers of twins who then choose to have another child primarily in order to experience this unique relationship with one baby. However, for couples with fertility problems it may be too late for them to have another pregnancy.

Siblings

A little-recognized problem arising from the arrival of multiples is the effect on other children in the family, particularly on the single toddler who has been the center of the family until suddenly displaced by an attention-attracting pair or trio. It has been shown that a sibling is likely to be more disturbed by the arrival of twins than of a single sibling and that behavior problems are more common in the older child[70]. Perhaps surprisingly Hay and colleagues[70] found that there was a greater increase in behavior problems amongst elder siblings who had experienced a longer gap before the arrival of the twins – a situation more likely to arise amongst subfertile couples.

In our experience at the MBF 'Supertwins Clinic' (for families with triplets and higher multiples) it is often the emotional response and behavior of the older sibling that is the cause of greatest concern to the parents. Stewart[71] found a high psychiatric morbidity, requiring specialist help, among the older siblings of seven families with quadruplets and higher births.

Triplets and higher-order births

Comprehensive information about the lives of families with triplets and higher-order births first became available from a series of linked surveys called the United Kingdom National Study of Triplets and Higher Order Births[26]. This study of over 300 families with higher-order birth British children born in 1980 and 1982–1985 covered medical and social aspects from the time of conception until the children were in school. The report demonstrated that the practical difficulties alone of looking after three babies at once are huge, even when all are healthy. Only with the greatest difficulty can a mother feed or transport them on her own. Many mothers cannot in practice cope with taking three babies together out of the home and so become effectively housebound and isolated. Meanwhile, the father may have to work longer hours to meet the significant extra cost of multiples.

Many parents, particularly those who have had many years to plan parenthood, become frustrated by their inability to give each child the individual attention that he or she deserves. The constant competition, fighting and noise can become wearing for the most tolerant. Even in those families with material resources and plenty of help, emotional stress, sometimes requiring psychiatric treatment, is not uncommon[72] (Box 8.2).

One mother in the MBF clinic, a nursery teacher, became deeply distressed by her inability to give each of her 2-year-old quadruplets the attention and stimulation that she knew they needed and deserved, and which she had been able to give with such commitment to her singleborn older son.

MULTIFETAL PREGNANCY REDUCTION

No clinician should regard triplets as an acceptable outcome of treatment for infertility and all should strive to reduce their incidence. Nor should multifetal pregnancy reduction (MFPR) ever be regarded as a solution to

---

Box 8.2

Comments by mothers of triplets

"I have regretted having three children. I thought for the first time that it was a high price to pay."

"The children saw me crying with fatigue. Sometimes I cannot stand up, physically or psychologically."

"Everything is done in a rush."

"Being super-efficient is not always easy. At the end of the day, I am completely broken."

Garel M, Salobir C, Blondel B. Psychological consequences of having triplets: a 4-year follow-up study. *Fertil Steril* 1997; 67: 1162–5

---

the problem even if it may in practice turn out to be the least worse outcome for some families.

There have now been numerous prospective non-randomized studies comparing pregnancy outcomes for MFPR twins with spontaneous twins and with triplets. A systematic review assessing effects of MFPR on fetal loss, preterm birth, perinatal mortality and infant morbidity showed no difference between the two groups of twins[73] and most have shown a better neonatal outcome for the surviving MFPR pair than the offspring of a continuing triplet pregnancy. It is clear that a randomized controlled trial could never be undertaken in view of the sensitivity and diversity of opinion on MFPR. These studies are so far limited to the first few years of life. The long-term psychological effect on the children is still to be established.

For many couples the overriding aim will always have been the safe birth of the one healthy child they originally sought. Their biggest concern has now become the health and welfare of any surviving babies or older children. With improvements in the care and long-term prognosis of preterm infants, an increasing number of obstetricians decline to reduce a triplet multiple pregnancy on medical grounds alone. The psychological effects that can result from the financial, practical and emotional stresses must also be taken into consideration. Nantermoz and colleagues[74] found, not surprisingly, that parents felt easier if they could perceive clinicians as carrying the main responsibility for the decision to reduce. Concern about any of these psychological aspects will vary greatly between couples and do not necessarily correlate with their socioeconomic status[75].

In a triplet pregnancy with a monochorionic pair, a couple considering MFPR face a particular dilemma. This is whether to sacrifice two (MZ) babies in order to preserve the fetus with the safer prognosis or to reduce the single fetus leaving two babies, each of whom is at higher risk of perinatal complications.

Some couples will think and feel MFPR to be contrary to their religious or moral values and this will be an important, although not necessarily crucial, factor in their decision. All carers, particularly counselors, therefore need some understanding of a couple's particular religion and culture[76].

Partners may themselves have difficulty in agreeing the right way forward. The father is often more worried by the increased risk of disability and the implications of having one or more children with special needs, whereas the mother is often more upset by the thought of being involved in the death of one of her babies.

The long-term implications need careful consideration. Should the parents tell the survivor or survivors about the fetal reduction or conceal it permanently? If the latter, it is essential that they disclose it to no one at all. Plainly all the medical carers need to be aware of this decision and this also raises problems of confidentiality for all staff currently involved but also those caring for the family through later treatments. One cost of parental secrecy is that the couple is inevitably deprived of the support of their friends and relatives.

For many of these couples with a higher-order pregnancy, this new dilemma of MFPR will add to a long history of stress with frustrated infertility treatments leading to low self-esteem and a feeling of recurrent failure[77]. Nevertheless, despite the emotional and other complications, it appears that the great majority who do proceed with a reduction feel ultimately that they had made the right decision[75,78].

Some parents will feel a profound bereavement and will understandably expect this to be respected. Some, of course, will prefer that others 'forget' what has happened.

There have been a number of follow-up studies reported on mothers following an MFPR[75,77–79]. All studies found that many of the mothers suffered emotionally with guilt and grief initially, but that few had serious problems after the first year. These results must, however, be viewed with caution. The number of mothers declining to participate was high.

Should a fetal pregnancy reduction sometimes even be considered in twin pregnancies? Such a reduction might be seen as logical in view of the recognized greater risks to twins compared to singleborn children, the increased safety of the procedure and the fact that many women are now conceiving twins in their forties. Evans et al.[80] reported that an increasing number of couples were requesting such a reduction and reviewed their own experience. Most clinicians, however, are very reluctant to destroy a potentially healthy twin unless there are serious medical maternal indications. However, some have now suggested that the good outcome in twin-reduced pregnancies should at least provoke discussion as to whether the procedure is justified more often than it is currently practiced[80]. A complex debate has opened. Some argue that if the alternative would be a termination of the whole pregnancy, a reduction to one would be preferable.

However, many single surviving twins are opposed, following their own deeply felt loss of their own twin. For them the bereavement of the survivor should be the overriding consideration.

COST OF MULTIPLE BIRTHS

The price of multiple births can clearly be high for both the parents and for the children themselves. However, a considerable price has also to be paid by the health and social services for the extra burden imposed by the multiple pregnancy and its outcome.

The cost of obstetric care of a multiple pregnancy is inevitably high. Preterm infants add a huge burden to the neonatal services through their extra technical, pharmaceutical and staffing requirements[81]. Furthermore, high multiples often use up most or all of the limited number of available neonatal intensive care cots. If the preterm delivery of triplets or quadruplets is expected in a hospital those cots must be kept free, thereby preventing the admission of ill singleton babies.

The average financial cost of neonatal care for a twin infant has been estimated to be 13 times that for a singleton. A triplet costs 41 times more and a quadruplet 77 times more than a singleborn infant. This means that, for the neonatal care alone, the infants from a quadruplet pregnancy will cost 308 times more than the infant from a singleton pregnancy[82].

Comparing the cost of IVF infants with those spontaneously conceived until the end of the neonatal period, Koivurova et al.[83] found a 1.3-fold increase for singleborn and 1.1-fold for twins.

Inpatient costs during the first 5 years were over twice as great for a twin child and five times for a triplet[84]. Inevitably the drain on the health services continues in later years. The children are more likely to have special needs and these will require ongoing pediatric care and other therapies as well as special education.

Some understanding of the costs of these can be derived from studies of low-birth-weight children in general. It has been shown that the health care up to 8 years of a low-birth-weight (< 2000 g) child costs, on average, five times as much as that of a child with normal birth weight. For a disabled low-birth-weight child the cost was 17 times greater. The total cost of health care and education up to the age of 8 years for a low-birth-weight child who survived with a long-term disability was four times that of a low-birth-weight child with normal development and nine times that of a normal birth-weight control[85]. Similarly, Petrou[86] found that the cumulative cost of hospital inpatient admissions incurred during the first 10 years of life was over four times as great in children born at less than 28 weeks' gestation than in those born at term. There are extra costs to social services of providing practical and emotional support to these families as well as the greater financial costs to the families[87].

ATTITUDE TO MULTIPLES

It is not surprising that couples who desperately want children often leap at the seemingly ideal prospect of having two or more children at the same time, and would underestimate the problems. For many the economic pressures to avoid further IVF treatments are a major factor, particularly in those countries, such as the UK and USA, where most ART still has to be funded by the couples themselves.

Early studies found that many couples considered twins a desirable out-come and some said they would even be happy at the prospect of triplets. Gleicher et al.[88] in the USA found that 67% of couples undergoing infertility treatment would 'love to have twins' and less than 10% would have been 'upset to have twins'. Indeed, 50% would not have been upset to conceive triplets. Similarly, Murdoch[89] in the UK found that 69% considered that twins would be the ideal outcome of their treatment. In the one study that distinguished the views of each partner, male partners were no less enthusiastic about having twins than their female partners[90].

However, more recent studies with higher response rates have found that couples may be given pause when they understand better the implications of a multiple pregnancy[90,91]. Grobman et al.[91] found that although most infertile couples initially wished to conceive twins their desire was affected by careful explanation of the probabilities of specific perinatal complications. This group was also much less positive than those in previous studies about having triplets.

Nevertheless, many couples are still eager to have twins. In another recent study[92], 20% of infertile couples said they would still prefer twins to a single baby. However, a high proportion were not aware of many of the risks of a twin pregnancy. Those with less knowledge were more likely to desire multiple births, as were the nulliparous and those who had had a longer duration of infertility. Perhaps surprisingly, those of younger age and of lower income were also keener to have twins, perhaps having in general less understanding of the risks involved, or being influenced by the public recognition that twins so often produce.

PREVENTION OF MULTIPLE BIRTHS

Inevitably most couples will have little knowledge of either infertility treatment or indeed of multiple births. They may well have difficulty in absorbing the barrage of information provided.

More clinicians providing treatment for infertility now appreciate the many medical and psychosocial disadvantages resulting from a twin conception, let alone that of a higher multiple. Nevertheless, there are still many who appear not to take sufficient account of the increased morbidity for both mother and children and the much higher perinatal mortality. Many more fail to give adequate thought to the stress that multiple-birth children can cause to a family.

Single embryo transfer is the only way to ensure that higher-order births are avoided and that the incidence of twins is substantially reduced. This undeniable fact appears to be much more readily accepted in some countries than others. What dictates this widely differing practice? Education and commerce are two factors to consider. For couples who must pay for their own treatment, there is clearly huge pressure on the clinician to produce a pregnancy in as few cycles as possible, whereas in Scandinavia, where treatments are government funded, patients are likely to be prepared to take the route most likely to produce a healthy child even if several extra (free) attempts are required.

Even when information on multiples is readily available, many clinicians take time to accept the implications for their practice. Despite the necessary knowledge and clear guidelines from the British Fertility Society and the Royal College of Obstetricians and Gynaecologists it was only when the UK's regulatory body – the Human Fertilisation and Embryology Authority – decreed that a maximum of two embryos should be transferred in women under 40 that the practice became widespread.

RESEARCH NEEDED

Despite the increasing awareness about the special problems associated with multiple births for both the children and their families, steps to halt the epidemic are still slow[5]. Many areas require further study not only to provide further information about the consequences of infertility treatments (Box 8.3) but also to ensure that those who do have twins and triplets receive the support and help they need[93].

Box 8.3

Areas for further research

Follow-up studies of iatrogenic twins and triplets

(a) Neurodevelopmental

(b) Psychological and emotional

(c) Psychosocial effects on family

(d) Long-term psychosocial consequences to parents and children following multifetal pregnancy reduction

Analysis of zygosity and chorionicity of multiple births following all forms of ovulation induction and assisted reproductive technology

The impact on the health-care services

(a) Financial cost

(b) Other resources (e.g. staff and cots)

(c) Effect on other patients

Patient information on multiple births

(a) Quality of information given to patients

(b) Feedback from patients – what do they wish they had known?

(c) How realistic were their expectations and in what way did they differ?

REFERENCES

1. Imaizumi Y. Trends of twinning rates in ten countries, 1972–1996. Acta Genet Med Gemellol 1997; 46: 209–18
2. Kiely JL, Kiely M. Epidemiological trends in multiple births in the United States, 1971–1998. Twin Res 2001; 3: 131–3
3. Macfarlane A, Blondel B. Demographic trends in Western European countries. In: Blickstein I, Keith LG, eds. Multiple Pregnancy. Epidemiology, Gestation and Perinatal Outcome. Abingdon, UK: Taylor and Francis, 2005: 11–21
4. Office of National Statistics. Series FM1 no. 31. Multiple Births, 2005
5. Fauser BCJM, Devroey P, Macklon NS. Multiple birth resulting from ovarian stimulation for subfertility treatment. Lancet 2005; 365: 1807–26
6. Loos R, Derom C, Vlietinck R, Derom R. The East Flanders Prospective Twin Survey (Belgium): a population-based register. Twin Res 1998; 1: 167–75

7. Blickstein I, Baor L. Multiple Births in Israel. In: Blickstein I, Keith LG, eds. Multiple Pregnancy. Epidemiology, Gestation and Perinatal Outcome. Abingdon, UK: Taylor and Francis, 2005: 48–50

8. MacGillivray I, Sampier M, Little J. Factors affecting twinning. In: MacGillivray I, Campbell DM, Thompson B, eds. Twinning and Twins. Chichester: John Wiley, 1988: 67–98

9. Derom C, Derom R. The East Flanders Prospective Twin Survey. In: Blickstein I, Keith LG, eds. Multiple Pregnancy. Epidemiology, Gestation and Perinatal Outcome. Abingdon, UK: Taylor and Francis, 2005: 39–47

10. Human Fertilisation and Embryology Authority. The HFEA Guide to Infertility and Directory of Clinics. London: HFEA, 2005

11. Kallen B, Finnstrom O, Nygren KG, et al. Temporal trends in multiple births after in vitro fertilisation in Sweden, 1982–2001: a register study. Br Med J 2005; 331: 382–3

12. Imaizumi Y. A comparative study of zygotic twinning and triplet rates in eight countries, 1972–1999. J Biosoc Sci 2003; 35: 287–302

13. Bryan E, Denton J, Hallett F. Zygosity Determination. Facts about Multiple Births. London: Multiple Births Foundation, 1997

14. Bamforth F, Machin G. Why zygosity of multiple births is not always obvious: an examination of zygosity testing requests from twins or their parents. Twin Res 2004; 7: 406–11

15. Ooki S, Yokoyama Y, Asaka A. Zygosity misclassification of twins at birth in Japan. Twin Res 2004; 7: 228–32

16. Jain V, Fisk NM. The twin–twin transfusion syndrome. Clin Obstet Gynecol 2004; 47: 181–202

17. Adegbite AL, Castille S, Ward S, et al. Prevalence of cranial scan abnormalities in preterm twins in relation to chorionicity and discordant birth weight. Eur J Obstet Gynecol Rep Biol 2005; 119: 47–55

18. Lopriore E, Nagel HT, Vandenbussche FP, et al. Long-term neurodevelopmental outcome in twin-to-twin transfusion syndrome. Am J Obstet Gynecol 2003; 189: 1314–19

19. Sutcliffe AG, Sebire NJ, Taylor B, et al. Outcome for children born after in-utero ablation therapy for severe twin-to-twin transfusion syndrome. Br J Obstet Gynecol 2001; 108: 1–5

20. Derom C, Derom R. Placentation. In: Blickstein I, Keith LG, eds. Multiple Pregnancy. Epidemiology, Gestation and Perinatal Outcome. Abingdon, UK: Taylor and Francis, 2005: 157–67

21. Blickstein I. Estimation of iatrogenic monozygotic twinning rate following assisted reproduction: pitfalls and caveats. Am J Obstet Gynecol 2005; 192: 365–8

22. Spandorfer SD, Rosenwaks Z. The phenomenon of monozygosity in iatrogenic pregnancies. In: Blickstein I, Keith LG, eds. Multiple Pregnancy. Epidemiology, Gestation and Perinatal Outcome. Abingdon, UK: Taylor and Francis, 2005: 214–17

23. Milki AA, Jun SH, Hinckley MD, et al. Incidence of monozygotic twinning with blastocyst transfer compared to cleavage-stage transfer. Fertil Steril 2003; 79: 503–6

24. Blickstein I, Jones C, Keith LG. Zygotic splitting rates following single embryo transfers in in-vitro fertilization: a population-based study. N Engl J Med 2003; 348: 2366–7

25. Miura K, Niikawa N. Do monochorionic dizygotic twins increase after pregnancy by assisted reproductive technology? J Hum Genet 2005; 50: 1–6

26. Botting BJ, Macfarlane AJ, Price FV, eds. Three Four and More. A Study of Triplet and Higher Order Births. London: HMSO, 1990

27. Alexander GR, Salihu HM. Perinatal outcomes of singleton and multiple births in the United States 1995–1998. In: Blickstein I, Keith LG, eds. Multiple Pregnancy. Epidemiology, Gestation and Perinatal Outcome. Abingdon, UK: Taylor and Francis, 2005: 3–10

28. Liu C, Blair E. Predicted birthweight for singletons and twins. Twin Res 2002; 5: 529–37

29. Blickstein I. Normal and abnormal growth in multiples. Semin Neonatol 2002; 7: 177–85

30. Koivurova S, Hartikainen AL, Sovio U, et al. Growth, psychomotor development and morbidity up to 3 years of age in children born after IVF. Hum Reprod 2003; 18: 2328–36

31. Ombolet W, De Sutter P, Van der Elst J, et al. Multiple gestation and infertility treatment: registration, reflection and reaction: the Belgian project. Hum Reprod Update 2005; 11: 31–4

32. Fitzsimmons BP, Bebbington MW, Fluker MR. Perinatal and neonatal outcomes in multiple gestations: assisted reproduction versus spontaneous conception. Am J Obstet Gynecol 1998; 179: 1162–7

33. Olivennes F, Kadhel P, Rufat P, et al. Perinatal outcome of twin pregnancies obtained after in vitro fertilization: comparison with twin pregnancies obtained spontaneously or after ovarian stimulation. Fertil Steril 1996; 66: 105–9

34. Dhont M, De Sutter P, Ruyssinck G, et al. Perinatal outcome of pregnancies after assisted reproduction: a case control study. Am J Obstet Gynecol 1999; 181: 688–95

35. Lambalk CB, van Hooff M. Natural versus induced twinning and pregnancy outcome: a Dutch nationwide survey of primiparous dizygotic twin deliveries. Fertil Steril 2001; 75: 731–6

36. Moise J, Laor A, Armon Y, et al. The outcome of twin pregnancies after IVF. Hum Reprod 1998; 13: 1702–5

37. NassarAH, Usta IM, Rechdan JB, et al. Pregnancy outcome in spontaneous twins versus twins who were conceived through in vitro fertilization. Am J Obstet Gynecol 2003; 189: 513–18

38. Bernasko J, Lynch L, Lapinski R, et al. Twin pregnancies conceived by assisted reproductive techniques: maternal and neonatal outcomes. Obstet Gynecol 1997; 89: 362–72

39. Hurst T, Lancaster P. Assisted Conception in Australia and New Zealand 1999 and 2000. Assisted Conception Series no 6. Sydney: AIHW, 2001

40. Pinborg A, Loft A, Schmidt L, et al. Neurological sequelae in twins born after assisted conception: controlled national cohort study. Br Med J 2004; 329: 311

41. Petterson B, Nelson KB, Watson L, et al. Twins, triplets and cerebral palsy in Western Australia in the 1980s. Br Med J 1993; 307: 1239–45

42. Topp M, Huusom LD, Langhoff-Roos J, et al. Multiple birth and cerebral palsy in Europe: a multicenter study. Acta Obstet Gynecol Scand 2004; 83: 548–53

43. Glinianaia SV, Pharoah PO, Wright C, et al. Fetal or infant death in twin pregnancy: neurodevelopmental consequence for the survivor. Arch Dis Child Fet Neonat Ed 2002; 86: F9–15

44. Yokoyama Y, Shimizu T, Hayakawa K. Prevalence of cerebral palsy in twins, triplets and quadruplets. Int J Epidemiol 1995; 24: 943–8

45. Stromberg B, Dahlquist G, Ericson A, et al. Neurological sequelae in children born after in-vitro fertilization: a population-based study. Lancet 2002; 359: 461–5

46. Keith LG, Goldman RD, Breborowicz G, et al. Triplet pregnancies in women aged 40 or older: a matched control study. J Reprod Med 2004; 49: 683–8

47. Oleszczuk JJ, Keith LG, Oleszczuk AK. The paradox of old maternal age in multiple pregnancies. Obstet Gynecol Clin North Am 2005; 32: 69–80

48. Garel M, Blondel B. Assessment at 1 year of the psychological consequences of having triplets. Hum Reprod 1992; 7: 729–32

49. Garel M, Salobir C, Lelong N, et al. Development and behaviour of seven-year-old triplets. Acta Paediatr 2001; 90: 539–43

50. Taylor EM, Emery JL. Maternal stress, family and health care of twins. Children and Society 1988; 4: 351–66

51. Thorpe K, Golding J, MacGillivray I, et al. Comparison of prevalence of depression in mothers of twins and mothers of singletons. Br Med J 1991; 302: 875–8

52. Tanimura M, Matsui I, Kobayashi N. Child abuse of one of a pair of twins in Japan. Lancet 1990; 336: 1298–9

53. Ostfeld BM, Smith RH, Hiatt M, et al. Maternal behaviour toward premature twins: implications for development. Twin Res 2000; 3: 234–41

54. Feldman R, Eidelman AI. Does a triplet birth pose a special risk for infant development? Assessing cognitive development in relation to intrauterine growth and mother–infant interaction across the first 2 years. Pediatrics 2005; 115: 443–52

55. Spillman JR. The role of birthweight in maternal–twin relationships. MSc Thesis, Cranfield Institute of Technology, 1984

56. Ellison MA, Hall JE. Social stigma and compounded losses: quality-of-life issues for multiple-birth families. Fertil Steril 2003; 80: 405–14

57. Ellison MA, Hotamisligil S, Lee H, et al. Psychosocial risks associated with multiple births resulting from assisted reproduction. Fertil Steril 2005; 83: 1422–8

58. Mahlstedt PP. The psychological component of infertility. Fertil Steril 1985; 43: 335–41
59. Klock SC. Psychological adjustment to twins after infertility. Best Prac Res Clin Obstet Gynaecol 2004; 18: 645–56
60. Glazebrook C, Sheard C, Cox S, et al. Parenting stress in first-time mothers of twins and triplets conceived after in vitro fertilization. Fertil Steril 2004; 81: 505–11
61. Pinborg A, Loft A, Schmidt L, Andersen AN. Morbidity in a Danish National cohort of 472 IVF/ICSI twins, 1132 non-IVF/ICSI twins and 634 IVF/ICSI singletons: health-related and social implications for the children and their families. Hum Reprod 2003; 18: 1234–43
62. Cook R, Bradley S, Golombok S. A preliminary study of parental stress and child behaviour in families with twins conceived by in-vitro fertilisation. Hum Reprod 1998; 13: 3244–6
63. Mushin D, Spensley J, Barreda-Hansen M. Children of IVF. Clin Obstet Gynecol 1985; 12: 865–76
64. Munro JM, Ironside W, Smith GC. Successful parents of in vitro fertilisation (IVF). The social repercussions. J Assist Reprod Genet 1992; 9: 170–6
65. Colpin H, Munter AD, Nys K, et al. Parenting stress and psychosocial well-being among parents with twins conceived naturally or by reproductive technology. Hum Reprod 1999; 14: 3133–7
66. Tully LA, Moffitt TB, Caspi A. Maternal adjustment, parenting and child behaviour in families of school-aged twins conceived after IVF and ovulation induction. J Child Psychol Psychiatry 2003; 44: 316–25
67. Bryan E. Twins with special needs. In: Sandbank AC, ed. Twin and Triplet Psychology. London: Routledge, 1999: 61–9
68. Lewis E, Bryan EM. Management of perinatal loss of a twin. Br Med J 1988; 297: 1321–3
69. Woodward J. The Lone Twin. Understanding Twin Bereavement and Loss. London: Free Association Books, 1998
70. Hay DA, McIndoe R, O'Brien PJ. The older sibling of twins. Aus J Early Child 1987; 13: 25–8
71. Stewart A. The long term outcome. In: Harvey D, Bryan E, eds. The Stress of Multiple Births. London: Multiple Births Foundation, 1991: 127–34
72. Garel M, Salobir C, Blondel B. Psychological consequences of having triplets: a 4-year follow-up study. Fertil Steril 1997; 67: 1162–5
73. Dodd J, Crowther C. Multifetal pregnancy reduction of triplet and higher-order multiple pregnancies to twins. Fertil Steril 2004; 81: 1420–2
74. Nantermoz F, Molenat F, Boulot P, et al. Implications de la réduction embryonnaire sur grossesse multiple: réflexions preliminaries. Neuropsychiatr Enfance 1991; 39: 594–7
75. Garel M, Stark C, Blondel B, et al. Psychological reactions after multifetal pregnancy reduction: a 2-year follow-up study. Hum Reprod 1997; 12: 617–22
76. Chertok I. Multifetal pregnancy reduction and halakha. Early Pregnancy 2001; 5: 201–10

77. McKinney MK, Tuber SB, Downey JI. Multifetal pregnancy reduction: psycho-dynamic implications. Psychiatry 1996; 59: 393–407

78. Schreiner-Engel P, Walther N, Mindes J, et al. First-trimester multifetal pregnancy reduction: acute and persistent psychologic reactions. Am J Obstet Gynecol 1995; 172: 541–7

79. Kanhai HHH, de Haan M, von Zanten LA, et al. Follow-up of pregnancies, infants and families after multifetal pregnancy reduction. Fertil Steril 1994; 62: 955–9

80. Evans MI, Kaufman MI, Urban AJ, et al. Fetal reduction from twins to a singleton: a reasonable consideration? Obstet Gynecol 2004; 104: 102–9

81. Mugford M, Henderson J. Resource implications of multiple births. In: Ward RH, Whittle M, eds. Multiple Pregnancy. London: RCOG Press, 1995: 334–45

82. Papiernik E. Cost of multiple pregnancies. In: Harvey D, Bryan E, eds. The Stress of Multiple Births. London: Multiple Births Foundation, 1991: 22–34

83. Koivurova S, Hartikainen AL, Gissler M, et al. Health care costs resulting from IVF: prenatal and neonatal periods. Hum Reprod 2004; 19: 2798–805

84. Henderson J, Hockley C, Petrou S, et al. Economic implications of multiple births: inpatient hospital costs in the first 5 years of life. Arch Dis Child Fet Neonat Ed 2004; 89: F542–5

85. Stevenson RC, Pharoah POD, Stevenson CJ, et al. Cost of care for a geographically determined population of low birthweight infants to age 8–9 years. II. Children with disability. Arch Dis Child 1996; 74: F118–21

86. Petrou S. The economic consequences of preterm birth during the first 10 years of life. Br J Obstet Gynaecol 2005; 112 (Suppl 1): 10–15

87. Petrou S, Aach T, Davidson LL. The long-term costs of preterm birth: results of a systematic review. Child Care Health Dev 2001; 27: 97–115

88. Gleicher N, Campbell DP, Chan CL, et al. The desire for multiple births in couples with infertility problems contradicts present practice patterns. Hum Reprod 1995; 10: 1079–84

89. Murdoch A. Triplets and embryo transfer policy. Hum Reprod 1997; 12 1(Suppl 1): 88–92

90. Child TJ, Henderson AM, Tan SL. The desire for multiple pregnancy in male and female infertility patients. Hum Reprod 2004; 19: 558–61

91. Grobman WA, Stout J, Klock SC. Patient perceptions of multiple gestations: an assessment of knowledge and risk aversion. Am J Obstet Gynecol 2001; 185: 920–4

92. Ryan GL, Zhang SH, Dokras A, et al. The desire of infertile patients for multiple births. Fertil Steril 2004; 81: 500–4

93. Bryan E, Denton J, Hallett F. Guidelines for Professionals: Multiple Births and their Impact on Families. London: Multiple Births Foundation, 2001

Chapter 9

Ethical aspects of the future health of ART children

Vic Larcher

In this chapter I consider some of the ethical issues that arise from the application of assisted reproductive technology (ART) and in particular their impact on the future health of those children. Both the range and application of ART have increased over the past two decades, with 1% of children in developed countries being conceived by ART[1]. Conception may now be technically possible for many infertile couples, providing them and others with a realistic possibility of fulfilling their dreams of having a child. However, the physical, emotional and developmental welfare of children born by ART is of significant importance, especially as this group are themselves growing to maturity. They may have questions about their origins and identity and how ART itself might have impacted on their current and future health and that of their own children.

Application of technology requires value judgements as well as scientific and technical skills. Society demands candor, transparency and accountability from professionals and clinicians[2] and an active involvement in decision-making, which is no longer the sole prerogative of clinicians. The public now has access to information previously only available to clinicians. The events described in the Bristol and Royal Liverpool children inquiries[3,4] may have eroded the trust in which clinicians were previously held. Good medical practice is more closely defined[5]. Media interest in health matters has increased, but not all reports are well balanced or critically objective, instead focusing on human-interest stories and controversy, conflict or scandal[6]. There is greater emphasis on the rights and liberties of individuals, increasingly backed by legislation and/or regulation of professional practice. When application of technology is limited by scarcity of resources, discussions on their allocation are difficult, controversial and not value free.

Unsurprisingly, contemporary medical practice involves ethical uncertainty regarding innovative or controversial treatments, who should receive them, and the process of fair decision-making. Tensions also arise from competing moral claims. In ART this involves balancing the rights and interests of would-be parents, potential children and the society that may support them. A particular concern is the extent to which the interests of potential children may be subsumed to the rights of putative parents and the increasing technological imperatives of ART. There are concerns that the interests of children in our society do not achieve the consideration they ought to receive[7]. It is therefore important to consider the ethical issues that arise in ART from the child's perspective, but without losing sight of the moral claims of parents or society or the moral basis of medicine.

THE MORAL BASIS OF MEDICINE

Clinicians have duties to save life, restore health and prevent disease[8]. The moral basis of all treatment is that it should provide more benefit than burden and should be based where possible on appropriate scientific evidence derived from ethically conducted research.

Clinicians also have a duty to respect the autonomy of their patients by respecting their right to as much self-determination as they are capable of exerting[9]. Importantly they should respect the human dignity of all patients regardless of their abilities. Hence, they should not use patients merely as a means of achieving their own professional goals without attempting to obtain appropriately informed consent.

Clinicians have responsibility to carry out both duties fairly and justly and with appropriate skill and care. They should act within the framework provided by national and, where relevant, international law[10].

The implications of these obligations for clinicians are clear. They should not do things to patients that might cause harm or could reasonably be foreseen to do so. Patients should not be deceived or manipulated into doing what clinicians believe to be best for them rather than being able to choose for themselves. To exercise this right they should be provided with adequate comprehensible information. The obligations to protect health and respect autonomy can and do conflict. Matters are even more complex when the interests of a third party, e.g. a child, are involved. The need to consider the welfare of future individuals provides further complexity. In normal circumstances the respect that is accorded to the principle of individual liberty or self-determination means that great importance is placed upon respecting the wishes, beliefs and preferences of those who are capable of expressing and acting upon them. But the duty to respect an individual's right to self-determination is not absolute, especially in circumstances when the exercising of that right places others at risk of serious harm. This is especially so when clinicians are asked to collaborate or collude with such choices. An individual's own moral rights do not absolve him/her of their duty to avoid harm to others.

Thus, parents of naturally conceived children have certain rights over the procreation and rearing of their children, but do not have a right to harm them by abuse, maltreatment or neglect. Although some parental behaviors during 'natural' pregnancies may attract moral censure, there is only limited legal protection for fetuses, because of the importance of respecting the autonomy of existing competent adults, as opposed to those as yet unborn (see below).

THE MORAL BASIS OF ART

The intention of ART is to achieve the safe conception and delivery of healthy children. ART is compatible with the moral basis of medicine in that it grants couples reproductive autonomy[11]. Because individual freedom is an important requirement for human flourishing, considerable justification is needed to override an individual's freely determined choices, irrespective of harm to the individual concerned or the personal views of others involved[12-14]. ART satisfies the principle of utility if it achieves the intended aim of maximizing the welfare, preferences and happiness of those involved. It also allows relief of the burden of infertility and the harms that that may accrue, and respects the human right to found a family.

Although there are strong prima facie moral arguments for ART, counter arguments that have some impact on the welfare of children conceived by it include the following[15].

ART is always wrong

Some embryos created by ART are not used and their right to life is violated (see below). The manipulations of embryos involved may themselves be harmful to future children. ART may raise the possibility of selecting characteristics not regarded as being morally significant, e.g. hair or eye color, stature and athletic prowess, thereby leading to eugenic manipulation of society (slippery slope argument). However, many natural pregnancies end in spontaneous abortion, despite the wishes of parents. Such events, whilst tragic, may represent the natural equivalent of embryo selection used in preimplantation genetic diagnosis (PGD). It may be that there is greater moral justification for the elimination of a severe genetic disease in a family than the harm caused by destroying the primitive embryo that bears it. The existence of a slippery slope does not mean that limits cannot be set or that general respect for the sanctity of life is lost.

ART is unnatural

Many ART techniques – e.g. intracytoplasmic sperm injection (ICSI), PGD – have no 'natural' counterpart but the same is true of a great deal of contemporary medical practice, e.g. the use of antibiotics to treat serious infection. Some natural selection and destruction of embryos occurs *in vivo*. Man has always sought to understand and control his environment, using technologies that harness natural laws or phenomena, without always attracting moral censure. Society condones some kinds of 'unnatural' behavior, e.g. same-sex partners, presumably because it does not regard such behavior as unethical or harmful.

It seems fair and just that 'unnatural' or 'extraordinary' techniques should be the subject of ethical analysis and debate, rather than summary rejection, or indiscriminate acceptance.

This does not mean that ART should not mimic natural events as closely as possible, for example in the attempted implantation of single rather than multiple embryos.

ART is against divine will: it involves playing God

Creation and destruction of embryos may offend religious sensitivities because of the view that technology usurps the role and purpose of the Creator. Those who provide ART may be at risk of desensitization to the importance of the sanctity of human life. However, those who practice ART often argue that, if anything, what they do imbues a greater respect for the nature of human life in all its diversity.

Other arguments against ART may have only an indirect impact on children's welfare. They include the harms that may follow the separation of the conjugal and reproductive functions of marriage and the assertion that ART damages women by controlling their reproductive choices and reinforcing archaic stereotypes about women's roles as child bearers and in child rearing.

However, ART is by its nature experimental and its long-term harms and benefits for the children it produces are not well defined. It follows that treatment should be used only if adequate safety has been shown by appropriate preclinical studies. The ethical considerations that should apply to research involving human subjects are well established[16]. In considering innovative treatments such as ART it may neither be possible nor desirable to place limits on research that may have unquantifiable benefits[17].

None of the foregoing arguments are definitive reasons for rejecting ART on purely moral grounds. There would need to be strong reasons for placing embargoes on technology that appears to confer more benefits than burdens to couples, and these would stem from harms to the child or the embryos that will form them.

There would seem, therefore, to be significant moral grounds for helping couples who wish to conceive a child by ART. However, desperation produced by infertility, or an inappropriate and unrealistic desire for children, may lead putative parents to take risks with their own health and that of their future child that professionals cannot sanction. Whilst professionals have a duty to collaborate with parents in their project to conceive they also have a duty and responsibility to the resultant child or children. Use of ART, as opposed to natural conception, is associated with prematurity, low birth weight and multiple pregnancies, all of which can have adverse effects on the health, development and educational prospects of the future child[16-20]. Additionally, ART increases the risk of birth defects independently of these factors[21]. Therefore, a cogent reason for controlling or rejecting ART relates to potential or actual harms to future children, the families who rear them and society in general. It is therefore important to consider the respective interests and claims of parents, society and children.

PARENTAL INTERESTS AND ART

Although there is wide public acceptance that parenthood should be regarded as a right, professional opinion is divided as to whether this should always be so[22,23]. The decision to become a parent may be irrational in that it is impossible to predict what the result of having children may be on the parents and others[24]. Some individuals may be unable to bear the responsibilities of parenthood, even if they wish to exert the rights that accompany it (Children Act 1989)[25]. There are no specific legal rights to parenthood even though the right to marry and found a family (European Convention on Human Rights) implies that the right to procreation is a strong one. Therefore, whilst we should not prevent couples from procreating without the strongest possible justification, there may not be a positive duty to assist them, e.g. by ART. An overemphasis on adult rights may be contrary to the needs of children[21].

Couples or individuals seeking ART presumably have similar motives for wanting children as do parents who conceive naturally[26]. Whilst some motives may be less morally acceptable than others, discomfort about motivation is usually an insufficient reason to infringe parental rights to natural reproductive choice[27]. Motivation is more likely to be examined in ART, in part because of the greater risks and resources involved.

Couples seeking ART might include the following: single and post-menopausal women, those infertile as a consequence of cancer treatment (in either partner), those sterile as a result of sexually transmitted disease, those with life-limiting illnesses, those with marital difficulties, and single-sex couples and couples with adverse psychosocial circumstances. There might be some in whom chances of success of ART might be so low as not to be a clinically worthwhile risk.

ART usually, but not always, involves clinicians, the exception being single-sex couples who use informal, unlicensed donation or even private surrogacy. Clinicians have duties to parents *and* future children. The moral acceptance of the duty to respect the autonomy of putative parents does not absolve clinicians of their duties to the child. There is no obligation to provide ART for all those who request it, especially if to do so compromises the health of parents or is not in the best interests of the future child.

Selection of individuals for ART is based on the medical status of parents and evaluation of the welfare of children produced. The UK Human Fertilisation and Embryology Act section 13(5) states 'a woman shall not be provided with treatment services unless account has been taken of the welfare of any child who may be born as a result of the treatment (including the need of that child for a father) and any other child who may be affected by the birth'[28]. This provision arguably discriminates against single and lesbian women and fails to respect their reproductive autonomy[22].

In many societies reasons for denying ART probably do reflect perceived family ideals rather than risk factors for the child[23]. Such objections may not be founded on morally relevant principles or a demonstration that there is harm to the growth and development of children when other compounding variables, e.g. education, are controlled. Indeed, positive social factors may compensate for some potentially poor developmental outcomes in children born by ART, and these may be absent in naturally conceived children. Some reasons for denying ART to putative parents do attract a level of agreement. They include ongoing substance abuse, domestic violence, severe marital disharmony and severe mental impairment. However, individuals who conceive naturally may also display these characteristics yet their freedom of reproductive choice remains unfettered until the point at which the child suffers or is likely to suffer from significant harm. Other parental characteristics that might limit access to ART are more controversial, for example maternal age and maternal weight. Decisions regarding eligibility for ART should be based on the extent to which the characteristic in question can be shown to have a significant impact on the physical, mental or emotional development of the child. Ascertainment of this is complex and requires detailed, thorough and long-term case controlled studies with adequate statistical power. In the meantime a strong case can be made for equality of access to ART in those societies where this can be offered. When access to ART is denied, the reasons must be clearly stated and based on acceptable and appropriate moral principles that should be applied equally and fairly to all relevant similar cases.

THE INTERESTS OF THE STATE AND REGULATION OF ART

State intervention in the right of adults to exercise natural reproductive choice can be justified only in the most extreme circumstances, e.g. the necessity to limit exponential population growth when resources cannot sustain it.

A moral obligation to assist infertile couples by providing ART is likely to produce significant competition for funding other with things that society may value, e.g. education, preventive medicine. Even if couples fund ART themselves, the State may still have a legitimate interest in the outcome, especially if the resulting child has disabilities requiring significant medical and educational support. States also have a duty to protect their citizens (including future children) from the harms associated with new technologies. More controversially they may seek to influence the type of society that evolves by favoring certain types of family unit over others.

THE INTERESTS OF FUTURE CHILDREN

Since the aim of ART is to produce healthy children, those who provide or fund it should consider the interests and welfare of these children and the embryos from which they are derived.

These issues are inevitably interwoven with legal and regulatory considerations. Because law confers status on some individuals but not others, there may be difficulties in protecting the interests of embryos and fetuses if they lack legal status. In contrast, biological parameters, e.g.

height or intelligence, are subject to variation amongst individuals and development over time. Pediatricians are used to dealing with such concepts and the inappropriateness of applying inflexible definitions of status or competency based on a single parameter, e.g. age. Pediatrics acknowledges the concept of gradually increasing moral status and slowly evolving capacities whose precise definitions may be blurred.

MORAL STATUS OF EMBRYOS

Since there are no significant moral justifications for killing a child it is important to determine at what stage in development from embryo to child it becomes a significant wrong to kill it. Hence the moral status accorded to embryos or the status that they possess is important. A pro-life approach argues that the embryo has the same identity as the child that it will become. Therefore, embryos have full moral status at conception, or at least after the point when twinning becomes impossible. The difficulty with this view is that it assigns the same status to a small group of cells as it does to a child and this seems intuitively wrong. If this view were adopted it would mean that techniques such as selective embryo reduction or PGD would be wrong even if failure to use them resulted in significant harm to the future child. A development of this view is to consider an embryo's moral status is a function of what it might become, so that killing it kills a potential child. However, eggs and sperm and even somatic cells (with cloning) are potential children. On an extension of the potential child argument, disposal of sperm or eggs is wrong[29], as is voluntary celibacy (which would prevent the generation of children)[30]. There appear to be few significant moral qualms about the disposal of somatic cells and most states prohibit their use in reproductive cloning.

A more pragmatic approach ascribes embryos and fetuses moral status in accordance with the extent to which they have properties that are associated with personhood. Since major criteria for personhood are consciousness, self-consciousness[31,32], rationality and an ability to interact with others, few would claim that embryos possess them. Whilst fetuses may feel pain from 24 weeks' gestation[33] this does not necessarily equate with consciousness, as it is generally understood.

Use of the above criteria may enable the setting of some absolute lower limits below which fetuses would not have significant moral status. However, the above criteria for personhood would set unrealistically high thresholds for the granting of moral status. Many 'normal' children and adults with learning difficulties would be excluded.

Society does grant babies (and fetuses?) certain moral status because of the good consequences that follow from this. Since babies clearly resemble humans and have an important social role it seems intuitively more wrong to kill a baby with severe learning difficulties than it does to kill an animal with the same level of personhood-satisfying criteria. Respecting the life of such children is an expression of humanity. The fact that ART may result in some children being born who will have educational or other difficulties is acceptable on these grounds because of their social importance.

Biologically it is possible to argue that moral status increases with fetal development. Early on, when moral status is low (but not absent) justification for killing would be less than it is at later stages of development. Killing an early fetus would therefore still be wrong but the degree of wrongdoing would be less and hence more easily justifiable. This pragmatic approach can be taken to justify most of the early embryo manipulations that form part of ART, including the selection and implantation of embryos with certain characteristics. It may even justify fetal reduction to avoid multiple pregnancies, though alternatives, such as the implantation of single embryos, would be ethically preferable.

COMPETING FETAL RIGHTS AND THE MATERNOFETAL RELATIONSHIP

There are practical difficulties with this pragmatic approach when maternal behavior threatens harm to the fetus. Normally there are strong moral and legal reasons for not interfering with the mother–child relationship. The law provides little protection for the rights of the unborn child (however conceived) even when maternal actions result in the death or serious handicap of the child[34] and has been reluctant to impose sanctions upon competent pregnant women who ignore or reject professional advice

Matters may be somewhat different when ART is involved, where the clinician's collaboration necessarily imposes a moral obligation to the future child. A mother whose baby has been damaged by her alcohol consumption has put her own self-destructive interests in drinking above those of her child. If she were a candidate for ART then it might be ethical to withhold it unless she indicated that she would stop drinking. In these particular and rare circumstances there may be justifications in infringing the woman's autonomy (albeit for self-destructive urges) and privacy for the sake of her baby, since any potential harms of ART might be compounded by her action and therefore not be in the best interests of the future child.

BEST INTERESTS OF CHILDREN BORN BY ART

One element in considering the interests of the future child is to determine whether the couple in question are the most appropriate to rear a child. By analogy with adoption this may involve some assessment of parenting ability. However, in adoption the adoptive parents are not usually closely biologically related to the child, as is the case in ART. Hence ART couples usually, but not invariably, have greater affinity with their offspring than might be the case in adoption. Older or single parents, who might be excluded from adoption, do not necessarily make poor biological parents. In adoption the identity of the baby is the same whoever is chosen to adopt him or her; in ART the identity of the child differs according to who provides the gametes. The adoption analogy may therefore be inappropriate to decide which couples should be helped[35]. Some other mechanism is required to make decisions that are in the best interests of the child.

A more relevant question is whether it is better for a potential child to be born to this particular set of parents by ART or not to be born at all. This is especially important if some forms of ART are associated with risks of physical or cognitive disability. For clinicians to assist in the creation of children who will have significant risks of disability may be just as wrong as it is for a woman to drink in pregnancy knowing that her baby will be harmed by her actions.

Robertson has argued that a higher incidence of birth defects associated with ART does not justify banning it[27,36]. Without ART the child would not be born at all and it cannot be in a child's interest not to exist. Unless the child's life is so full of pain and suffering as to be worse than no life at all s/he has not been harmed by the technology that created him/her. Therefore, if the only alternative for the child is not to be born at all, then the person who has helped the child to be conceived has not injured him/her.

This argument supposes that those who do not exist have some interest in being born. However, it is difficult to see how preconceptual non-existence deprives a child of anything, or what interests they might have[37]. Since preconceptual non-existence can be neither good nor bad, a life with serious defects would be worse than such a state. Possible children can have interests in the sense that we ought to act in a way that promotes their welfare if they were to be born. Hence it has been argued in connection with genetic diseases that children ought not knowingly be conceived 'when there is a high risk of transmitting a serious defect [of a sort that would deny them] a normal opportunity for health'[38].

It may be only severe forms of disability that should be considered worse than no existence (e.g. permanent vegetative state), and that some conditions, for which prenatal screening and termination are offered (e.g. Down's syndrome), should be excluded because they are compatible with a reasonable life[39].

Prenatal screening for such disabilities is therefore objectionable because of the offence it causes to people with disabilities who are currently living (the 'expressivist objection')[40]. But, whilst discrimination against children with disabilities who currently exist or who will be born naturally is wrong, this does not mean that avoiding their creation is wrong. The obligation not to harm disabled people by offending them may not trump others' rights to have their reproductive autonomy respected. The abortion of fetuses with disability is accepted, presumably because moral justification of acting early in pregnancy overcomes any stricture against killing. It may also be morally wrong to ask parents to care for a child that they do not want. However, this latter argument may not give enough weight to the child's interests and too much to parental autonomy.

Second, it is possible to hold simultaneously the views that screening for disability can be performed *and* that existing disabled people should receive all the care and social support that they need.

Third, the expressivist objection seems to imply that it is wrong to seek to prevent any form of disability or have it cured or reduced. This seems counterintuitive and incompatible with the moral basis of medicine.

It may be preferable that there were no or minimal risk of disability, but in the specific circumstances of individual parents there may be no choice. If clinicians do not help such parents it may be inferred that they do so for at best unethical and at worst eugenic reasons. They should, however, use techniques that minimize the risk of disability if the latter exist and have been validated.

The interests of the potential child from that child's own perspective are more difficult to ascertain, since substituted judgements made on behalf of someone who may never exist can be considered absurd. But this does not prevent potential parents entertaining hopes and aspirations on their future child's behalf, however irrational they may seem[24]. A potential child might prefer creation by ART even with the risk of serious disability than not to have existed at all. Alternatively, the child might not want to be born with a serious disease or defect of the sort that would deny him or her a normal opportunity for health.

It is therefore unclear whether a potential child might come to the view there was a right not to be born at all rather than to be born with a disability or to be born with a level of disability that would permit a reasonable life. There would also be difficulties in deciding whether embryos positive for adult-onset disease should be screened out, since the potential child would have been denied 40 years of healthy life. However, it does seem clear that some degrees of disability can be regarded as existence that is worse than death or at least a living death. Severe disability of this nature could be characterized by a life that was so full of pain and suffering, limited in span, and lacking in meaningful social interactions that no reasonable person would want to live it. Moreover, parental capacity to cope with a child with disability differs enormously. Some parents may regard the care of a disabled child as a positive experience but others might feel that it involves sacrifices that they are unable to make. Respect for parental autonomy should not grant parents the right to reject a child for trivial or morally irrelevant reasons.

Many of these considerations involve what may be termed quality of life judgements. Life may have limited value depending on the extent to which certain qualities associated with flourishing (e.g. health, choices, social interaction) are lacking or diminished. Because these qualities are intangible and incommensurable, it has been argued that decision-making in medicine should be based on the clinician's offer of the most appropriate evidence-based treatment and the patient's consent or refusal to it, whilst still allowing considerable discussion[41].

CONSENT TO ART

Valid consent is required for all medical treatment and intervention. To be ethically and legally valid, consent should be freely obtained, given by a person who is competent to do so, and based on adequate information[42]. Parental anxiety about infertility and its implications may render their choices less free and limit their competence. Competent individuals must be able to understand and retain information, believe that it applies to them or their particular circumstances, and use it to make the decision in question[43].

A particular issue with ART lies in the information standards that ought to be used. The information that a reasonable and responsible body of medical opinion might disclose is inadequate because it fails to respect autonomy sufficiently. Information that a reasonable person in the patient's circumstances might want to make the decision in hand is scarcely sufficient when innovative treatment is proposed, which may have unquantifiable harms and benefits. Arguably, those who make complex decisions on behalf of others should, in order to fulfil their duty properly, have access to information, which that particular person might want for himself or herself. It could certainly be argued that a relevant standard of information for ART is that which each individual couple want for themselves or their future child. Moreover, there is a clear duty to consider the amount of information that the future child might wish that his parents had received in making their decision to conceive him. There is some legal basis for this increased information standard[44]. It might be reasonable that those who are likely to provide future care for the child might be involved at an earlier stage than is current practice, because of their knowledge of child health.

PREIMPLANTATION GENETIC DIAGNOSIS

PGD relies on the ability to produce embryos from single sperm, to culture and perform microsurgery on them and to enhance small quantities of DNA for diagnostic purposes and the reliable exclusion of relevant conditions[45]. Unsuitable embryos can be discarded and suitable embryo(s) implanted. It is particularly useful for couples with a known genetic risk – usually determined by the birth of a previously affected child – who may have already had a termination and who wish to be sure of an unaffected pregnancy[46]. It provides alternatives to gamete donation, adoption or prenatal diagnosis and termination. Its moral justification depends on accepting that it is ethical to carry out experiments on pre-embryos, knowing that some will be destroyed (see above).

Research using PGD techniques has demonstrated the difficulty of extrapolating data from embryo experiments in animals to humans and problems associated with some techniques of egg recruitment. Such research has had scientific benefits and has implications for the risks of ART to future children[47].

PGD carries risks that include exposure of embryos to chemicals, physical effects, removal of blastomeres and direct damage from culture media *in vitro*. Although numerous children have been born following PGD there are few specific reports on outcomes and especially those involving a control population. It would be particularly upsetting if a technique designed to reduce chances of serious genetic disorders produced other damaging effects that raised ethical concerns about its use.

PGD gives parents considerable reproductive autonomy, but it is not clear whether PGD can or should be limited to only genuine medical purposes to prevent serious genetic disease. It can also be used for screening (for conditions other than the 'risk' one) and sex selection for other than genetic indications, e.g. family balancing (in those families who had a genuine desire to do so). There are concerns that its future use might involve selection of less morally relevant characteristics by those who can afford to do so. Families might also wish to use PGD to select children who will have their own genetic condition (e.g. deafness, achondroplasia) because they hold strong positive views about their own condition and the wrong of discriminating against it. They may believe that a 'normal' child will suffer more discrimination and stigma than one with their condition. Whilst colluding with parents respects their autonomy, this arguably fails to take adequate account of the interests of the future child. If PGD does carry greater risks than natural conception there may be insufficient justification for its use in these particular circumstances[47].

PGD has also been used to create 'savior siblings' who are a tissue match for an existing child with a life-limiting condition for which marrow or stem cell transplantation offers the only effective cure, e.g. Fanconi anemia, thalassemia major. PGD alone provides a new unaffected child, a tissue match and cure for the sick child, thereby achieving the most positive outcomes of the alternatives and satisfying the utilitarian calculus[48]. One objection, contested by such parents, is that the creation of a new life to save an existing child uses the new baby merely as a means to save another. There may also be unforeseen harms, and the altruism of the created child cannot be assumed. Nonetheless, regulatory authorities have accepted PGD for serious genetic disease and other life-threatening but non-genetic illness, e.g. leukemia.

PGD can also be used to select embryos free from adult-onset disease, e.g. Huntington's chorea, but ethical dilemmas arise when parents stipulate non-disclosure of their own state. Discarding embryos that have many potential disease-free years is problematic. Even more so is the inability to tell parents if screening shows that they are unaffected, because disclosure would enable them to conceive by natural means and avoid the hazards and expense of ART. In this case the best interests of the future child would surely override parental right to confidentiality and non-disclosure.

The moral justification for PGD lies in the benefits and respect for reproductive autonomy it allows families. However, the risks to future children are unclear and need to be defined by appropriate research.

THE PREVENTION OF MULTIPLE PREGNANCIES DUE TO ART

Children conceived by ART have more complications than those conceived by conventional means. Whilst singletons born after ART have a greater risk of low birth weight and multiple birth defects, multiple pregnancy, and especially twin pregnancy, is an even greater risk factor[18,19]. Multiple pregnancies have a higher rate of perinatal mortality and morbidity and neurodevelopmental and psychological sequelae. There are increased immediate and long-term costs associated with multiple deliveries, especially when associated with prematurity or low birth weight.

A single pregnancy would represent as nearly as possible the natural state. Advances in technology have enabled single embryo transfer (SET) to achieve acceptable pregnancy rates in certain circumstances. Prospective parents need to be informed of the risks of multiple gestations and the harms that this may produce for the children concerned[49]. They may not be competent to make informed choices because of overwhelming emotions and lack of availability of sufficient objective information on outcomes. Professionals have a duty to enhance parental competence by education and counseling, but have no obligation to provide treatment that they do not believe to be in the best interests of couples or children.

The number of embryos may be reduced *in vivo* by non-selective fetal reduction, which reduces the risks associated with multiple pregnancies but at the expense of other risks, e.g. spontaneous abortion. Although fetal reduction may be ethically justified, it would be better avoided by implanting single or a small number of embryos[49].

Increasing success rates for SET suggest that previous practices of multiple embryo transfer can no longer be ethically justified on risk–benefit grounds. However, only 9% of IVF cycles in the UK in 2002–03 involved SET as opposed to over 70% involving two[50]. This highlights the need for audit and review of practice especially in the area of innovation or rapidly changing treatments. The obligations to review and modify practice and keep up to date stem from the moral basis of medicine.

GAMETE DONATION, ANONYMITY AND CHILDREN'S RIGHTS

The rights of children are increasingly recognized. The UN Convention on the Rights of the Child sets out the rights of children to health, to family life, to knowledge of their own identity and to having their voices heard (in accordance with their age and understanding) in matters that concern them[51]. Application of the Convention has implications for children conceived by ART, especially with regard to identity. Despite a societal shift to greater transparency and accountability that finds expression in a trend to non-anonymous gamete donation, in practice relatively few ART children know of their method of conception or the identity of their gamete donor. The reasons for this are several[52]:

(1) Donors wish to retain their right to privacy and wish to disclose little personal information;

(2)   Introduction of non-anonymous donor schemes has led to a decline in donor numbers;

(3)   Disclosure of the method of conception infringes a family's right to personal privacy and may have adverse effects on intrafamilial relationships;

(4)   Although societal stigma of illegitimacy has lifted, the child may suffer stigmatization and discrimination if their origin were known;

(5)   In contrast to adopted children, children conceived by ART may not suffer from genealogical bewilderment and psychological harms[34], and may have family and social relationships that do not differ from those of naturally conceived children[53]. However, difficulties in obtaining appropriate research data occur because of the anonymity which has surrounded gamete donation until recently.

However, arguments that disclosure is not in the child's best interests virtually all take adult perspectives and, in the context of children with life-limiting illness, may be significantly discordant with the child's view[54].

There are other good reasons why children should be told of their origins. Knowledge of one's own identity is essential to human wellbeing; to be denied such knowledge may be harmful. Irrespective of any harmful outcome, donor offspring have a right to be told the truth about their conception and origins, because of a general duty of truth telling. Donor offspring should not be the only group in society specifically denied the right to know the identity of their parents. Secrets, especially when revealed, may produce unhappiness, rage and confusion both in childhood and in adult life[55]. There is the intuitive argument that if children are not told they are somehow the recipients of injustice and wrongful treatment.

The nature of much ART makes it possible to conceal the nature of the child's conception, with over 70% of heterosexual couples deciding not to tell their offspring how they were conceived. Even when mature children were allowed identifying information about their gamete donor, 89% of parents had not informed them of the circumstances of their conception[56]. In contrast, same-sex couples did plan to tell their child; 40% wanted the identity of the donor to be registered[52].

Despite significant support for non-anonymized donation and free access by sufficiently mature children, adults may still control the flow of information. In the UK, children over 18 can be told whether they were the products of licensed treatment and can obtain some information about their donor, but must first suspect that they were conceived by ART, and, if they live with heterosexual couples, this seems unlikely. Warnock's suggestion that the child's birth certificate could indicate whether the conception was by donation has not been implemented[57].

A further option allows ART participants (both donors and recipients) to choose between anonymous and non-anonymous donation programs. This would give parents greater choice over what they told their children and maintain donor numbers, but fails to grant children the right of access to information.

REGULATION OF ART

One response to the ethical challenges of ART is to impose prohibitions reinforced by law; but this approach is inflexible and inappropriate, since it fails to reflect the complexity of competing moral claims. An alternative is some form of regulation that responds to complex scientific information, technological imperatives, diverse moral views, lack of clear public consensus, insufficient health and safety data, and intuitive as opposed to foundational ethical argument[58]. Any regulatory system therefore needs to be comprehensive, well informed and responsive to the pace of technical change, but operate within an agreed ethical framework and have an educational role. Importantly it should have powers to ensure that the interests of those who receive ART and those conceived by it are adequately considered and met. Such a system needs to be transparent, accountable and as free as possible of political constraints[59].

Although such systems are in place, they may not provide adequate safeguards for the welfare of children and not all centers that offer ART have clearly defined protocols to address this.

FOLLOW-UP OF CHILDREN BORN BY ART: REGISTRATION

One of the key factors in considering the welfare of children born by ART is knowledge of its consequences for their physical health, neurological development and emotional wellbeing. Studies such as the EPICure study have begun to define these outcomes for very-low-birth-weight infants and may have important consequences for the delivery of neonatal intensive care[60,61]. Similarly, the long-term effects of cancer treatment have been recognized and used to counsel patients and families and modify treatments to produce improved survival with less morbidity.

ART is associated with a higher risk of multiple pregnancies, premature births and birth defects than natural conception, but the latter have only recently been defined by meta-analysis. Further large, adequately powered, case controlled studies are necessary to define causative mechanisms, associated factors and health-care needs. It is a requirement of good medical practice that clinicians critically evaluate their practice. If the purpose of ART is the production of healthy children, this is a relevant and appropriate outcome measure for audit. Follow-up may benefit individual children because it enables early identification of health-care or neurodevelopmental problems and allows treatment and support to be given. It also respects children's rights and enables clinicians to fulfil their duty of care. There may be more widespread benefits from follow-up, if it provides data that define the safety of various types of ART. Such data can be used to counsel future parents in making informed choices about treatment options.

However, follow-up for research purposes may have adverse consequences that cannot be foreseen and it is a matter of parental choice as to whether they become involved. Obtaining suitable control data may be difficult. The need for information has to be set against the duty to respect the right for privacy over personal health information that should not be in the public domain.

A confidential register of information on individual children could be kept, but data collection needs to be comprehensive and universal to be useful. Increasingly, data collection and storage require consent and ethical approval; both may be difficult to obtain[54]. However, it is possible to compile and analyze information whilst retaining confidentiality, for example by encoding data and giving the responsibility of holding the codes that link the data to an identifiable person to someone other than those responsible for entering the data or analyzing it[62].

Since pediatricians will be concerned with follow-up it seems reasonable that they, with fertility specialists, might have a greater role in the counseling of putative parents.

CONCLUSIONS

ART extends the ability of would-be parents to exercise their reproductive autonomy[12,13], but at some costs to the children created. Therefore, future needs of children should be considered in any extension or new application of ART. This process involves complex value judgements on behalf of an individual who does not yet exist, has no legal status and no voice. Moreover, treatment decisions may be made in circumstances where obtaining properly informed consent may be difficult. It is important that the future child has an advocate and, with an increasing proportion of children conceived by ART, perhaps this is an appropriate role for pediatricians.

It may be impossible to decide whether it is better for a particular child to be born or not[39]. The future child would certainly wish (were s/he able to do so) that his or her parents received appropriate information about the risks of future harm and the actions to be taken to prevent or reduce them. S/he would wish that those providing ART had safety as their paramount concern and that a fair balance had been struck between his/her rights and those of his/her parents.

The conclusions reached here do not preclude research with embryonic stem cells or with pre-embryos. However, when the intention becomes the production of a healthy child, techniques should be used that maximize the chances of successful conception but with minimal risk to the child. In the short term some negotiated compromise of parental autonomy may be necessary to define better risk/benefit consequences for children, including those that might arise from a right to know their origins. This approach would be consistent with the moral principles of medicine and is likely to be in accord with the best interests of children and what they might wish for themselves.

REFERENCES

1. Sutcliffe AG. Health risks in babies born after assisted reproduction. Br Med J 2002; 324: 117–18
2. Warnock M. A national ethics consultation. Br Med J 1988; 297: 1626–7
3. Bristol Royal Infirmary. The Inquiry into the Management of Care of Children Receiving Complex Heart Surgery at the Bristol Royal Infirmary. London: HMSO, 2001
4. The Royal Liverpool Children's Hospital. Inquiry Report 2001. London, HMSO, 2001
5. General Medical Council. Good Medical Practice. London: GMC, 2001
6. Seale C. Media and Health. London: Sage, 2002
7. Aynsley-Green A, Baker M, Burr S, et al. Who is speaking for children and adolescents and for their health at the policy level? Br Med J 2000; 321: 229–32
8. Callahan D. An international project of the Hasting Center. The goals of medicine setting new priorities. Hasting Center Rep 1996; 26 (Suppl): 52–4
9. Doyal L. Needs, rights and the moral duties of clinicians. In: Gillon R, ed. Principles of Healthcare Ethics. London: Wiley, 1993: 217–30
10. Chantler C, Doyal L. Medical ethics: the duty of care in principle and practice. In: Powers M, Harris N, eds. Clinical Negligence. London: Butterworth, 2000
11. Doyal L. Infertility counselling and IVF. The moral and legal background. In: Jennings S, ed. Infertility Counselling. Oxford: Blackwell, 1995: 191–204
12. Mill JS. On Liberty. Harmondsworth: Penguin Books, Reprinted 1987: 68

13. Harris J. Rights and reproductive choice. In: Harris J, Holm S, eds. The Future of Reproduction. Oxford: Clarendon Press, 1998

14. Strong C. Ethics in Reproductive and Perinatal Medicine. New Haven, CT: Yale University Press, 1997

15. Hope T, Salvulescu J, Hanceuck J. Reproductive medicine. In: Medical Ethics and Law – the Core Curriculum. London: Churchill Livingston, 2003: 115–31

16. World Medical Association. Declaration of Helsinki (as amended by 52nd WMA General Assembly Edinburgh 2000). France: WMA Ferney-Voltaire, 2000

17. Nuffield Council on Bioethics. Animal to Human Transplants: The Ethics of Xenotransplantation. London: Nuffield Council on Bioethics, 1996

18. Lambert RD. Safety issues in assisted reproduction technology. Hum Reprod 2002; 17: 3011–15

19. Schieve LA, Meikle SF, Ferre C, et al. Low and very low birth weight in infants conceived with use of assisted reproductive technology. N Engl J Med 2002; 346: 731–7

20. Helmerhorst FM, Perquin DAM, Donker D, Keirse MJNC. Perinatal outcome of singletons and twins after assisted conception: a systematic review of controlled studies. Br Med J 2004: 328: 261

21. Hansen M, Baver C, Milne E, et al. Assisted reproductive technologies and the risk of birth defects – a systematic review. Hum Reprod 2005; 20: 328–38

22. Maclean M. Parenthood should not be regarded as a right. Arch Dis Child 2005; 90: 782–3

23. Boivin J, Pennings G. Parenthood should be regarded as a right. Arch Dis Child 2005; 90: 784–5

24. Bennett R. Human reproduction: irrational but in most cases morally defensible. J Med Ethics 2004; 30: 379–80

25. The Children Act. London: HMSO, 1989

26. Langdridge D. Problems of indeterminacy and deontology. Hum Reprod 2000; 15: 502–4

27. Robertson JA. Children of Choice: Freedom and the New Reproductive Technologies. Princetown, NJ: Princetown University Press, 1994: 75–6

28. Human Fertilisation and Embryology Act. London: HMSO, 1990

29. Singer P. Technology and procreation: how far should we go? Technol Rev 1985; Feb/Mar: 23–30

30. Singer P, Kuhse H. The ethics of embryo research. Law Med Health Care 1987; 14: 133–8

31. Tooley M. Abortion and Infanticide. Oxford: Oxford University Press, 1983

32. Singer P. Practical Ethics, 2nd edn. New York: Cambridge University Press, 1993

33. Anand KJS, Hickey PR. Pain and its effects in the human neonate and fetus. N Engl J Med 1987; 317: 1321–9

34. Re MB. An Adult: Medical Treatment. 1992. 2 FLR. 426 CA

35. Shenfield F, Steele SJ. What are the effects of anonymity and secrecy on the welfare of the child in gamete donation? Hum Reprod 1997; 12: 392–5

36. Robertson JA. Procreative liberty and the control of conception, pregnancy and childbirth. In: Baruch EF, Adamo J, Seager AF, eds. Embryos, Ethics and Women's Rights: Explaining the New Reproductive Technologies. New York: Harvard Press, 1988: 179–94

37. Cohen CB. 'Give me children or I shall die'. New Reproductive Technologies and Harm to Children. Hasting Center Report 26, No 2. 1996: 19–27

38. Purdy LR. Genetic disease: can having children be immoral? In: Buckley J Jr, ed. Genetics Now. Ethical Issues in Genetics Research. Washington, DC: University Press of America, 1978: 25–39

39. Savulescu J. Is there a right not to be born? Reproductive decision making, options and the right to information. J Med Ethics 2002; 28: 65–7

40. Edwards SD. Disability, identity and the 'expressivist objection'. J Med Ethics 2004; 30: 418–20

41. Downie RS. The value and quality of life. J R Coll Physicians Lond 1999; 33: 378–81

42. Montgomery J. Health Care Law. Oxford: Oxford University Press, 2002: 227–48, 437–39

43. Re C [1994] 1 All. ER 819

44. Rogers v Whittaker [1992]. 175. CLR 479

45. Taylor AS, Braude PR. Preimplantation diagnoses of genetic disease. In: Studd J, ed. Progress in Obstetrics and Gynaecology. London: Churchill Livingstone, 1994: 1–20

46. Bickerstaff H, Flinter FA, Yeang CT, et al. Clinical application of preimplantation genetic diagnoses. Hum Fertil 2001; 4: 24–30

47. Braude PR. Preimplantation genetic diagnoses and embryo research – human developmental biology in clinical practice. Int J Dev Biol 2001; 45: 607–11

48. Boyle R, Savulescu J. Ethics of using preimplantation genetic diagnoses to select embryos for stem cell donor for an existing person. Br Med J 2001; 323: 1240–3

49. Pennings G. Avoiding multiple pregnancies in ART. Hum Reprod 2000; 15: 2466–9

50. www.hfea.gov.uk

51. United Nations Convention on the Rights of the Child. General Assembly of the United Nations Convention on the Rights of the Child (1989). London: HMSO, 1996

52. Frith L. Gamete donation and anonymity: the ethical and legal debate. Hum Reprod 2001; 16: 818–24

53. Golombek S, Breweays A, Giavazzi MT, et al. The European Study of assisted reproduction families: the transition to adolescence. Hum Reprod 2002; 17: 830–40

54. Bach JR, Campagnolo DI, Hoeman SI. Life satisfaction of individuals with Duchenne's Muscular Dystrophy using long term mechanical ventilatory support. Am J Phys Med Rehabil 1991; 70: 129–35

55. McWhinnie A. Gamete donation and anonymity. Should offspring from donated gametes continue to be denied knowledge of their origins and antecedence? Hum Reprod 2001; 16: 807–17

56. Gottlieb C, Lalos O, Lindblad F. Disclosure of donor insemination to the child: the impact of Swedish legislation on couples' attitudes. Hum Reprod 2000; 15: 2052–6

57. Warnock M. The good of the child. Bioethics 1987; 2: 141–55

58. Caulfield T, Knowles L, Meslin EM. Law and policy in the era of reproductive genetics. J Med Ethics 2004; 30: 414–17

59. Blackburn E. Biothetics and the political distortion of biomedical science. N Engl J Med 2004; 350: 1379–80

60. Wood NS, Costeloe K, Gibson AT, et al. The EPICure study: associations and antecedents of neurological and developmental disability at 30 months of age following extremely preterm birth. Arch Dis Child Fetal Neonatal Ed 2005; 901: F134–40

61. Vohr BR, Wright LL, Dusick AM, et al. Neurodevelopmental and functional outcomes of extremely low birth weight infants in the National Institute of Child Health and Human Developmental Neonatal Research Network 1993–4. Pediatrics 2000; 105: 1216–26

62. Ingelfinger JR, Drazen JM. Registry research and medical privacy. N Engl J Med 2004; 350: 1452–3

Chapter 10

Conclusions

Alastair G Sutcliffe

This book represents a contemporary review of a changing field. There have now been many sincere efforts to evaluate the ultimate outcome of assisted reproductive technology (ART), namely the health of children born with the help of these treatments.

It remains true today that the prima facie risk of ART is the birth of twins, triplets or more, despite recent efforts towards single embryo transfer (SET) in the Scandinavian countries[1]. Hopefully, the precedent set in Scandinavia will become more and more widespread via legislation and ultimately, if that legislation does not work, particularly in countries where 'personal freedom is a maxim'. . . by litigation. In the chapter written by Elizabeth Bryan and Jane Denton there is a depressing series of facts concerning the risks to twins and particularly to triplets, whether or not they are born after ART per se. This chapter should be heeded especially by the fertility specialist reader or any parent who reads this book who is deceived by the false logic that replacing more than one embryo will somehow increase the overall pregnancy rate. There are a number of trials ongoing which will further clarify this issue (which one accepts is not absolutely black and white for elderly mothers). Caution should be conveyed to any parent considering exposing themselves to the risk of ART twins by noting that at most of the presentations given by the editor throughout the world on the topic of this book at least one parent has approached him with a sad story that they had had IVF twins or triplets and one of these children had cerebral palsy or worse.

In the first chapter of the book written by Professor Simpson we are enlightened as to the common difficulties which studies of ART outcome produce[2]. Ultimately, families cannot be *obliged* to take part in studies; however, it is possible for countries to mandate that certain key information be collected about these ART births which can be obtained in order to establish critical facts concerning the health of children at birth. Here the Scandinavian countries have been particularly effective but are limited by their small populations. Thus, in order to obtain meaningful data, they have often had to carry out analyses over a considerable period of time which will thus distort any messages from those data[3]. Nonetheless, there is an emerging field of evidence from studies performed in different parts of the world to show that families who use ART are more likely to have a child with congenital anomalies[4-7]. However, this risk, when allowing for all potential confounders, the nature of which are discussed in considerable detail by Professor Wennerholm, Professor Bergh and Dr Kurinczuk and colleagues in their chapters, is only about 1.2–1.5 times that of the background population, thereby raising an important philosophical point for the practicing pediatrician to draw to the attention of the reader. If a child is born with a congenital anomaly after ART, the family will immediately ask whether the process of ART was implicated and furthermore, if that child has something rare such as Angelman syndrome[8], it may be easy to be dismissive and say that this disorder is very rare. Nonetheless, it is not at all rare for that particular family, and it can have a profound effect on their personal life.

What families commonly do not ask, which perhaps they should, is what is the genetic makeup of my family that increases my risk of having a child with a congenital anomaly? This remains one of the outstanding questions concerning pediatric outcome, namely, that it is still unclear with the best available evidence whether the risk is solely as a result of the genetic makeup of those families who are having ART. From this book it is not possible to reasonably conclude (perhaps surprisingly in the case of intracytoplasmic sperm injection, ICSI) that there is a direct effect of the processes of ART that results in the congenital anomalies. Nonetheless, it is now reasonably convincing that Angelman syndrome and Beckwith–Wiedemann syndrome[9] appear to be disorders for which there is a plausible process by which ART may result in their development. For example, the syndromes may arise owing to aberrant imprinting as a result of the differing culture media used. That evidence is also supported from the work by Professor Reik[10] and others regarding culture media experiments in animal models. These matters need to be further explored[11].

Continuing the commentary on congenital anomalies it also appears that there is a high risk of monozygotic twins after ART which is unexplained[12]. However, as stated above in terms of congenital anomalies as a whole, we can now say with some confidence that there is a higher risk which is a little above that of the background population. When large countries such as Britain, Germany or the United States (in terms of population) validate the efforts by Scandinavian countries to address these issues, the final picture will emerge and hopefully will be reported in a future edition of this book.

Moving on to the perinatal period after ART, again one remains unconvinced that there are any distinguishing factors between *in vitro* fertilization (IVF), ICSI and/or embryo cryopreservation outcomes. However, it has been substantially confirmed by studies performed throughout the world that children who are singletons born after ART are more likely to be premature and more likely to be of low birth weight[13–15]. This of course particularly applies to twins, triplets or higher-order births as stated at the beginning of this concluding chapter.

The largest detailed study of children assessed beyond the newborn period at age 5 years[16–18] reveals some interesting facts concerning the health and wellbeing of ART children. First, the boys born after ICSI were more prone to needing urological surgery[17], and this is perhaps not surprising, since it has long been recognized that urological abnormalities result in reduced fertility and those fathers who are requiring ICSI, at least for its initial indications, were more likely to pass on whatever urological abnormalities they had to their male offspring. This logically also brings up the issue of future fertility[19], and here it is fair to say that children born after ICSI would appear to be at higher risk of subfertility as adults by virtue of the fact that some of them have Y chromosome deletions, such as DAZ-L or YRRM deletions, which had been passed on by fathers by way of their Y chromosome to their male children. However, to make the quantum leap to the statement that they will be subfertile is a different matter altogether, as technology is changing fast in this area of medical advancement.

Studies of neurodevelopment of children born after ART allowing for confounders (such as prematurity) do not show any evidence that they are per se at increased risk of neurological/neurodevelopmental problems[16,18,20–22]. Whilst there have been suggestions of increases in cerebral palsy[23], this is confounded by the fact that these children may have been from twin pregnancies in which one twin had died, or by the fact that the information gathered was by relatively inaccurate or poor proxies and thus cannot be relied on to make a definitive statement about this. Overall, the literature suggests that ART children are developmentally normal providing they have no specific risk factors which would be the same for naturally conceived children. This is an important and reassuring piece of information which could be passed to any family who are considering having ART of whatever kind.

This brings us to the family relations and effect on rearing of their ART children. It has taken 25 years for a substantive study[16] to be published which looked at a large number of families not from a single center and investigated how they were getting on in relationships between members of the family, how their children were perceived, how parents perceived their children, and so forth. Although early work by Golombok et al.[24], Gibson et al.[25] and McMahon et al.[26] have alluded to these possibilities, the recent study produced by Professor Barnes and teams across European cultures[16] confirms that families who had an IVF- or ICSI-conceived child experienced parenting in a very positive manner but enjoyed work less. However, this needs to be confirmed at a later age and indeed, as this book is going to press, I am informed of further follow-up work in Belgium (Professor Ponjaert, personal communication) suggesting that this tendency to have these positive images of your child as an ART parent, in comparison to naturally conceived children, remains at child age 8 to 9 years. As Professor Barnes pointed out, however, if this 'rosy' image represented in any way denial in the sense that the families claim to enjoy work less than naturally conceiving families, then those same ART parents may resent this 'self sacrifice' at a later stage and this could have a less positive implication for the child's personal identity and sense of self-worth, as they grow up. This remains to be seen.

This brings one to the ethical side of ART and a comment. As a population of individuals, ART-conceived children will become a significant stakeholder group as adults, representing anything up to 3% of the population[27] in some Western countries. If they have long-term risks due to the exposure to ART, their view of that risk being taken by their parents and fertility specialists could be very different from those who have undergone and been involved in the treatment process from the beginning. Therefore, we would have to be cautious and consider setting up prospective studies of new variants of ART such as blastocyst transfer, whilst also acknowledging that ART is here to stay. It is a salient fact that the journal *Pediatrics*, on reviewing all the inventions from the previous century, regarded IVF[28] as one of the greatest inventions of mankind. To those involved in this treatment process, either as fertility specialists, fertility nurses, or counsellors, it is certainly an honor for those skilled teams to be able to help families with this most personal of needs. One hopes that this book is a worthwhile reference source for these professionals and that the success of such techniques will continue to improve so that ultimately everyone who wishes to have a child will be able to have that right.

REFERENCES

1. Kallen B, Finnstrom O, Nygren KG, Olausson PO. Temporal trends in multiple births after in vitro fertilization in Sweden, 1982–2001. Br Med J 2005; 331: 382–3

2. Simpson JL. Registration of congenital anomalies in ART population: pitfalls. Hum Reprod 1996; (Suppl 4): 81–8

3. Wennerholm UB, Bergh C, Hamberger L, et al. Incidence of congenital malformations in children born after ICSI. Hum Reprod 2000; 15: 944–8

4. Bergh T, Ericson A, Hillensjo T, et al. Deliveries and children born after in-vitro fertilisation in Sweden 1982–95: a retrospective cohort study. Lancet 1999; 354: 1579–85

5. Ludwig M, Katalanic A. Malformation rate in fetuses and children conceived after ICSI: results of a prospective cohort study. RBM online 2002; 5: 171–8

6. Hansen M, Kurinczuk J, Bower C, et al. The risk of major birth defects after intracytoplasmic sperm injection and in vitro fertilization. N Engl J Med 2002; 346: 725–30

7. Bonduelle M, Liebaers I, Deketelaere V, et al. Neonatal data on a cohort of 2889 infants born after ICSI (1991–1999) and of 2995 infants born after IVF (1983–1999). Hum Reprod 2002; 17: 671–94

8. Ludwig M, Katalanic A, Gross S, et al. Increased prevalence of imprinting defects in patients with Angelman syndrome born to subfertile couples. J Med Genet 2005; 42: 289–91

9. Maher ER, Brueton LA, Bowdin SC, et al. Beckwith–Wiedemann syndrome and assisted reproductive technology (ART). J Med Genet 2003; 40: 62–4

10. Reik W, Dean W. DNA methylation and mammalian epigenetics. Electrophoresis 2001; 22: 2838–43

11. Sutcliffe AG, Peters CJ, Bowdin S, et al. Assisted reproductive therapies and imprinting disorders – a preliminary British survey. Hum Reprod 2006; 21: 1009–11

12. Derom C, Derom R, Vlietinck R, et al. Iatrogenic multiple pregnancies in East Flanders, Belgium. Fertil Steril 1993; 60: 493–6

13. Wennerholm UB, Bergh C, Hamberger L, et al. Obstetric and perinatal outcome of pregnancies following intracytoplasmic sperm injection. Hum Reprod 1996; 11: 1113–19

14. Wennerholm UB. Cryopreservation of embryos and oocytes: obstetric outcome and health in children. Hum Reprod 2000; 15 (Suppl 5): 18–25

15. Wennerholm UB, Bergh C. Outcome of IVF pregnancies. Fetal Matern Med Rev 2004; 15: 27–57

16. Barnes J, Sutcliffe AG, Kristoffersen I, et al. The influence of assisted reproduction on family functioning and children's socio-emotional development: results from a European study. Hum Reprod 2004; 19: 1480–7

17. Bonduelle M, Wennerholm UB, Loft A, et al. A multi-centre cohort study of the physical health of 5-year-old children conceived after intracytoplasmic

sperm injection, in vitro fertilization and natural conception. Hum Reprod 2005; 20: 413–19

18. Ponjaert-Kristoffersen I, Tjus T, Nekkebroeck J, et al. Psychological follow-up study of 5-year-old ICSI children. Hum Reprod 2004; 19: 2791–7

19. Fisher-Jeffes LJ, Banerjee I, Sutcliffe AG. Parents' concerns regarding their ART children. Reproduction 2006; 131: 389–94

20. Sutcliffe AG, D'Souza SW, Cadman J, et al. Outcome in children from cryo-preserved embryos. Arch Dis Child 1995; 72: 290–3

21. Sutcliffe AG, Taylor B, Saunders K, et al. Outcome in the second year of life after in vitro fertilisation by intracytoplasmic sperm injection: a UK case–control study. Lancet 2001; 357: 2080–4

22. Sutcliffe AG, Saunders K, Mclachlan R, et al. A retrospective case–control study of developmental and other outcomes in a cohort of Australian children conceived by intracytoplasmic sperm injection compared with a similar group in the United Kingdom. Fertil Steril 2003; 79: 512–16

23. Pinborg A, Loft A, Schmidt L, et al. Neurological sequelae in twins born after assisted conception: controlled national cohort study. Br Med J 2004; 329: 311

24. Golombok S, Brewaeys A, Cook R, et al. The European study of assisted repro-duction families: family functioning and child development. Hum Reprod 1996; 11: 2324–31

25. Gibson AT, Ungerer JA, McMahon C, et al. The mother–child relationship fol-lowing in vitro fertilization (IVF): infant attachment, responsivity and mater-nal sensitivity. J Child Psychol Psychiatry 2000; 41: 1015–23

26. McMahon C, Ungerer JA, Tennant CC, Saunders DM. Psychosocial adjustment and the quality of the mother–child relationship at four months postpartum after conception by in vitro fertilization. Fertil Steril 1997; 68: 492–500

27. Friedler S, Mashiach S, Laufer N. Births in Israel resulting from in-vitro fertilization/embryo transfer, 1982–1989: National Registry of the Israeli Association for Fertility Research. Hum Reprod 1992; 7: 1159–63

28. Steptoe PC, Edwards RG. Birth after the reimplantation of a human embryo. Lancet 1978; 2: 366

Index